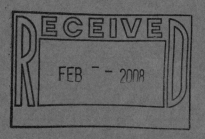

# ER
# Vet

PET ER
*Memoirs of an Animal Doctor*

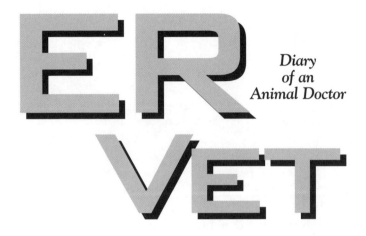

# ER VET

*Diary
of an
Animal Doctor*

2-8-08    George A. Porter

*To Karen —
Enjoy!
George A. Porter, D.V.M.*

HILLSBORO PRESS
Franklin, Tennessee

Printed in the United States of America

05    04    03    02    01        1    2    3    4    5

Library of Congress Catalog Card Number: 00-109651

ISBN: 1-57736-217-9

*Cover design by Gary Bozeman*


*Many cats featured in the illustrations are from Happy Tales Humane Society in Franklin, Tennessee (www.isdn.net/happytales/).*


HILLSBORO PRESS
PROVIDENCE HOUSE PUBLISHERS

238 Seaboard Lane • Franklin, Tennessee 37067
800-321-5692
www.providencehouse.com

This book is dedicated to my loving wife, Marilyn.
Marilyn has been my support throughout life
and emits an enthusiasm
that stimulates me in my endeavors.
She has always been available to assist me
in any manner at any time.
Marilyn has assumed the responsibility
of raising our three sons in a Christian environment
to insure that they develop into mature Christian men.
This was done with little assistance from me
for I was mostly unavailable
due to my hectic veterinary practice.
Marilyn has insurmountable energy
and radiates her exuberance to all
that come in contact with her.
She has the ability to involve others
in her charitable work
and is loved by all—especially me.

# CONTENTS

**M**y previous book, *Pet ER*, contained vignettes about my life as a veterinary practitioner when I worked at six different hospitals during normal daylight hours and took emergencies at eleven hospitals at night, on weekends, and on holidays. This book, *ER Vet*, is about my experiences from 1970–1974 after I opened my own hospital, Marina Animal Hospital, in Redondo Beach. I worked the daylight hours exclusively at my own practice but continued to take emergencies at the other eleven hospitals, plus my own, for a grand total of twelve hospitals.

My three sons, Bradley Allen, Bartell George, and James Albert, grew older and developed into more able assistants during this period of time. (I refer to my sons by their middle names throughout the book.) My wife, Marilyn (Marna) continued her proficient responsibility of being an intermediary between the four answering services and myself for the numerous calls that continually seek emergency care. My family surrounded me with the necessary assistance of constantly being available and skilled in handling the incoming emergency calls. After I opened my own hospital, Marna was always on call and available to fill in for staff members whenever they were sick or on vacation.

With my own hospital now responsible for providing emergency care in off hours, I realized that I should also include in this book the daytime or regular hour emergencies that occurred; animals who are in critical need have problems during those hours as well. I have used the name Jo to describe my many very capable assistants at the reception desk, in surgery, as radiograph assistants, and as kennel help. For their devotion and support to the health and well being of my patients, I am grateful.

In the years that I practiced emergency medicine, all emergencies were taken at the hospital whose exchange called me. This meant a lot of travelling—especially at night. This is why Marilyn's assistance was so valuable for she knew where I was at all times and would relay calls to me saving me considerable time driving and enabling me to see the pets more quickly.

My emergency workload continued at about the same pace after Marina Animal Hospital opened. I was involved with about 125 emergencies a month, which included the treatment cases that I often took at various hospitals on Sundays and holidays. During the seven years of taking emergencies on a contract basis, almost ten thousand cases were seen.

I contemplated giving up emergency contract work as I was beginning to feel the wear and tear of working so many hours per day, week, and month. It was apparent that the need of my family for the presence of a husband and a father was becoming more important to me.

It must be noted that during the period of time I was taking these many emergencies, few hospitals had gas anesthetic machines like the ones I had grown accustomed to using while in school. Gas anesthesia provided a better and safer anesthesia compared to the commonly used intravenous methods at that time. To provide this better and safer anesthesia, I purchased an anesthetic machine and carried it in the trunk of my Mustang, which was fitted with styrofoam partitions. This machine went with me at all times; I became very proficient in assembling it and dismantling it whenever needed at the various locations where I took emergency cases.

# Acknowledgments

Irst and foremost I wish to thank my wife, Marilyn, for encouraging me as well as supporting me in my endeavor to write this book. Marilyn put up with me when I would cloister myself in the house and request that I not be interrupted. She had to pretend that I was not there, and that is difficult for a person who abounds in enthusiasm and exuberance.

My sons played a major role not only as characters in the book *ER Vet* but also in coming forth with reminders about the cases that had interesting situations but had slipped my memory. Brad, Bart, and Jim frequently would phone at anytime day or night and ask if I remembered a certain case. This was a great help in providing material for my writing.

My family also helped by editing the early drafts of *ER Vet*. Brad and his wife, Leslie, and Jim and his wife, Lorraine, scrutinized each chapter carefully for grammar and sentence structure. My computer with its spell check was of great assistance, also.

Providence House Publishers with Andy Miller at the helm needs to be recognized as well. Andy and his staff made numerous recommendations that enhanced the quality of this book. They helped me organize my thoughts and present them in a proficient manner.

I'm also grateful to the friendly staff of Happy Tales Humane Society at the Factory in Franklin, Tennessee, for allowing me to include pictures of their adorable cats that are available for adoption. Many of my clients also provided wonderful pictures of their dogs.

To all who helped me produce this book—family, friends, and professionals—I am indeed indebted. I must not overlook the value of my clients and their pets for without their unusual cases, their personalities, and the situations that occurred, this book would never have come to fruition.

# ER
## VET

# 1 -

## A FOIL CASE

I had finished the day at my Redondo Beach hospital and headed home. I pulled into the driveway and was greeted by my two oldest sons, Allen and George, and our German shorthair pointer, Greta. The boys had been playing "dog tennis." They used a tennis racket to hit the ball down the street and Greta would retrieve it and the show would continue. The boys had the habit of tiring of the exercise first. Greta would prefer to play the game twenty-four hours a day.

The boys returned to their game of dog tennis with Greta, and I went into our house. On the end of the kitchen counter was a brown bag—a sure sign that I should have kept my Mustang's engine running. The brown bag contained my sack dinner. This meant that an emergency was in store for me. Marna came into the kitchen and informed me that I needed to call the Hawthorne exchange. The operator connected me to the Linharts. The Linharts' dog, Jasper, had been hit by a car. Mr. Linhart had already left home with Jasper and was on his way to that hospital. I shed my coat and tie, donned a sweater, and headed for my Mustang. Marna came running out with my brown bag that we called a sack dinner. I was then on my way.

Mr. Linhart was waiting in his car when I arrived. Jasper was on the back seat motionless except for his eyes. He tried to focus on me when I looked through the car window. Mr. Linhart picked Jasper up and followed me into the treatment room and set him on the table.

Jasper needed to be stabilized as he was in shock and may have lost blood internally. He was skinned up all over but no profuse quantity of blood was noted. I started a saline and 5 percent dextrose solution intravenously. The steroid, solu-delta-cortef, was added to control shock. I pulled up a couple of stools while the two of us monitored Jasper.

Mr. Linhart was in tears and nearly in a mild state of shock. I got him a glass of cold water and he just sat there watching his pet and occasionally looking at me for some sign of encouragement.

In a few minutes Jasper started moving his tongue, which had been hanging out of his mouth. He pulled his tongue into his mouth, and it changed from a dry appearance to that of a moist one with the addition of his saliva. He now appeared more alert and even made a feeble attempt to raise his head. All of these were good signs and I related this to Mr. Linhart.

I suggested that some X rays should be taken while Jasper was still in a semi-conscious state. We needed to ascertain what damage might have occurred other than his right rear leg that was obviously fractured. I carefully picked Jasper up and carried him into the X-ray room while his master rolled the attached intravenous stand in at the same time. The radiograph indicated that his right rear leg was broken in mid-shaft just distal to the head of the femur. From that view, I was also able to see damage to the pelvis. Another X ray was taken to better determine the extent of the damage there. The acetabulum [socket] of the femur exhibited a fracture that indented the right side of the pelvic bone internally until it almost touched the left side. If left as it was in that position, this pelvic fracture would occlude the passage of any feces.

Jasper's mucous membrane color was gradually changing from a grayish color to a healthier pink. He was raising his head now and looking at his owner and responding to his owner's voice. We transported Jasper as we had before to the critical care ward. Another liter of solution was connected to the drip system.

We went to the front room and I entered Jasper's name and vital statistics (male Australian Shepherd, six years old) as well as Mr. Linhart's address and telephone number on the client/patient medical record card. Mr. Linhart said, "Jasper chased a cat across the street. A car missed the cat but struck Jasper squarely on the right hip and spun him around.

Fortunately he was knocked away from the car and was not run over. The driver stopped and offered to help and I thanked him. I did not know what to do until I called a hospital and your answering service told me where to take him after they had talked with your wife."

We chatted for a few minutes about drivers stopping when animals are injured. He appreciated the driver's concern. I explained to him that I was going to splint his dog's leg and try to temporarily align Jasper's pelvic fracture before I went home. Surgery would be done the next day and I asked him to phone the hospital in the morning and talk to the doctor in charge. "The doctor will fill you in on his surgery schedule." I planned to monitor Jasper for awhile and I promised to call Mr. Linhart and give him a report on the Australian Shepherd before I left for home.

I made some coffee, sat down, and ate my sack dinner. Jasper was looking brighter each time I checked him, but he was still very immobile. I placed Jasper again on the treatment table and fitted a temporary splint on his right leg to prevent the sharp ends of the femur from severing any blood vessels or nerves. Then I put on some examination gloves and was able to open his pelvic area sufficiently enough so that he could eliminate. The attending doctor would have an hour or two of surgery to perform in the morning.

I made out a cage card for Jasper, wrote "fracture case" on the surgery board, and then headed for home. Marna and I had a time for the boys to go to bed and, like all children, they always tried to extend it to the limit. My three sons were just being tucked in when I arrived. They had tried to wait up for me and it was now ten minutes past their designated bedtime. Each got a hug, and I heard their prayers. I turned out their lights and retired to the family room with Marna.

We were sitting there wondering if there was enough time in the day to warrant starting a fire in the fireplace when the telephone rang. Marna was in the kitchen preparing several cups of coffee. She was nearest the phone so she picked up the receiver. It was for me. The Manhattan Beach hospital operator was on the line and asked if I would talk to a Mrs. Todd about her female cat Fluffy.

I was connected directly to Mrs. Todd. Something strange was going on. Fluffy was drooling a lot and she was having trouble finding the cause. "First she hid under the bed and when I finally got her out, she slipped from my grasp and disappeared again into the other bedroom's closet. My two children were helping me and they started chasing Fluffy all over the house. She was now very spooked and was doing her best to evade all of us. The children were hyper and that didn't help matters either."

My first question was, "Is she confined now?"

"No."

"Do you have a cage for her?"

"Yes."

"Can you get her into the cage?"

"I don't know."

"Where is she now?"

"Behind the couch in the living room. She is so frightened now I am almost afraid to pick her up."

"Try putting the cage into a position at the end of the couch so that the door is open the way Fluffy is facing. Get the children out of the room and let your cat calm down a bit. When she is calm, reach over the back of the couch and gently encourage her to move forward until she enters the cage."

"You mean pick her up?"

"Not necessarily. Don't take a chance of getting scratched or bitten. When you get her confined in the cage, please call back."

I had no idea how long I would have to wait for the return phone call, so I went ahead and built the fire in the fireplace. Marna had coffee ready so we sat down to have a short evening's visit. Twenty minutes later the return call was made. Fluffy was under control. Mrs. Todd would meet me at the Manhattan Beach hospital as soon as possible.

She was waiting in the parking lot when I arrived. I went over to the car to carry the cage in. Mrs. Todd was sitting in the passenger seat with the cage on her lap and she introduced her neighbor to me who was behind the wheel. She had gone next door to see if his wife would sit with the children. "He would not think of having me drive to the hospital alone, so he brought me down in his car," she explained.

All four of us went into the exam room. I carefully lifted Fluffy from the cage. I saw a beautiful Persian cat with orange eyes who was soaked in slobber from her chin down. Even the insides of her paws were wet for she had been using them to try and rid herself of the profuse saliva that was still dripping from her mouth.

Fluffy watched me very attentively. I reached for her head to restrain her so that I could open her mouth. She would have none of that! Immediately she shook her head and cast saliva around the room. I changed tactics. I covered her head with a towel and then extracted her right front leg from beneath her cloth protection. Mrs. Todd secured her leg in the proper position. An elastic tourniquet was applied and some surital anesthetic was titered into her vein. Soon we felt her relax. I wiped the saliva from her face and opened her mouth. Between her teeth on the upper left dental arcade was a piece of aluminum foil tightly wedged between her teeth. The foil was approximately the size of a large postage stamp.

I needed two hands to remove the foil, so I applied a feline oral speculum to keep her mouth open. Mrs. Todd again assisted me by holding Fluffy's head at the proper angle. The foil was then easily removed. The side of her face was slightly abraded where she had been pawing at herself in hopes of removing that irritating foreign object. I gave the cat an antibiotic injection to avoid a skin infection and dispensed some ointment to apply to her face.

Mrs. Todd said, "I don't know where she got the foil. However, she does get into the trash on occasion." She thanked me as well as her chauffeur for our evening's efforts. As she was departing, I noticed a jar full of suckers on the counter, so I gave Mrs. Todd two for her children. She and her neighbor left and I did so after cleaning the premises.

When I got home, Marna was sitting by the fire in her bathrobe watching the embers. She thanked me for laying the fire even though I did not really have a chance to enjoy it. We spent the remainder of the evening together sipping coffee by the remaining glow.

# 2 –

# A LEAD PELLET

**T**he operator for the Palos Verdes hospital was on the phone. The person on her line was frantic and needed to talk to me immediately. I was connected without gaining any further information from the operator.

Mrs. Mapes was hysterical. Her cat, Radisson, had been badly injured and was hemorrhaging. I told her that I would meet her at that Palos Verdes hospital and instructed her to drive carefully. I left immediately without finishing my dinner for this was a stat case.

I had to drive further than Mrs. Mapes and she was holding Radisson in her arms at the hospital door as I pulled into the parking lot. She was patiently waiting for me with tears streaming down her face. I took her tortoise shell, short-haired female cat from her arms and headed for the treatment room. Radisson was comatose and very pale in color. It was easy to start an intravenous drip and I added solu-delta-cortef to the solution to counter shock. I controlled the bleeding on her right side by applying a gauze pressure pack and then snugly taping it to her abdomen with elastic tape.

I returned to my Mustang and brought in my gas anesthetic machine so I could administer oxygen to my critically injured patient. I passed Mrs. Mapes who was in the reception room and observed that she was so distraught that I felt she might pass out. After connecting the oxygen to the endotracheal tube that I had entubated, Radisson's color began to improve. I checked the refrigerator and found sixty milliliters of feline blood and commenced another drip in the opposite front leg.

I monitored Radisson for a few minutes and went out front to question Mrs. Mapes but she was unable to talk with me. She was in a trance, looking out into space. I called Marna to come down and lend a hand. Marna arrived shortly. Radisson was doing a little better. Mrs. Mapes was not a regular client at this hospital, so Marna questioned her enough to get the necessary information to fill out the client/patient record card. Mrs. Mapes had no idea what had happened. I asked Marna to call Mrs. Mapes's husband and have him come down to take my distraught client home. We were informed that Mr. Mapes was a pilot and out of town. Eventually Marna obtained the information she needed to contact one of her neighbors who volunteered to come down with her husband. In no time at all her neighbors were walking in the front door of the hospital.

I still couldn't get any valuable history from Mrs. Mapes, so I proceeded on my own after she gave me a nod of approval. An X ray was taken. Considerable fluid, very likely blood, was evident in Radisson's abdomen. A lead pellet was the most distinguishing feature noted on the radiograph. I gently unwrapped the pressure pack on her abdomen and there was a pronounced hole in the right side that indicated the entrance of the pellet.

I clipped the hair from her ventral midline and scrubbed her down with surgical soap and then painted the area with an antiseptic solution. The wound on her side was prepared in the same manner. I carried my patient into surgery pushing the gas machine ahead of me. Marna followed pulling the intravenous drip stand with the attached solutions.

I opened the abdomen ventrally with an incision through the linea alba [ventral midline] and to my dismay found ingesta [partially digested food] floating free in a mass of blood. This indicated a perforated bowel. Marna went out front with this information and came back with the "go ahead and do all I can" instructions. I located perforations near the bowel so both sides of that lesion were clamped off with Doyne forceps. Next, I lavaged [rinsed] the wound several times with a sterile solution to eliminate much of the ingesta and blood that was hampering my vision. I was able to locate the blood vessels that were causing the hemorrhaging and clamped them off. The pellet was difficult to locate but was soon in the grasp of my forceps. I removed it and placed it on the counter. Marna rinsed it off and then took it out front to show everyone what had caused the injury.

Correcting the lesion in the bowel required immediate attention. When the bowel resection was completed, I carefully placed the bowel back into the abdomen into its normal position. The abdomen was again lavaged several times and antibiotics were placed into the abdominal cavity to avoid any possibility of peritonitis [inflammation of the abdomen]. No further bleeders were noted so the ventral midline incision was closed. Radisson was turned so that her right side was exposed and the entry port of the pellet was sutured.

The oxygen supply was continued by itself for no anesthetic was needed during the entire procedure. I replaced the intravenous drip solution with a 5 percent solution of saline and dextrose at a rate of one drop every fifteen seconds. Radisson's eyes were still glazed over, but the color of her mucous membranes was better than when I had initially seen her. Marna had prepared a cage and padded it well with several towels. Together we carefully moved the cat into intensive care with both the oxygen supply and the drip connected to her. I closed the surgery door so that the mess would not be offensive to my client or her neighbors, washed up, put on a clean smock, and went out front to give a progress report.

Mrs. Mapes was more composed now after being comforted by both Marna and her friends. Mrs. Mapes said that Radisson had been found as a wayward kitten wandering in the Radisson Hotel parking lot—hence her name. Mrs. Mapes had gone out into her laundry room and noticed her cat resting upon a stack of soiled clothes. "I thought that she was just taking a nap for that is where she likes to rest. About an hour later, I went out to do the wash. She was still there. I tried to coax her off so I could do the laundry. She didn't move. I picked her up to get to the clothes. She was limp. A large blood stain was on the clothes where she had been. My hands had blood on them, too. I called you immediately." Mrs. Mapes went on to explain that, "Radisson comes and goes through a cat door, so that is how she gained entrance to the house."

"Radisson could have been hit by the pellet even two blocks away and made it back to the house before the loss of blood weakened her so much she could not move anymore," I exclaimed. "Fortunately she found comfort resting in a place where you would likely find her. You can be thankful of that!"

The entourage was escorted to the intensive care ward where they all took a look at Radisson. Felines, when they are recovering from an anesthetic, frequently flex their paws. Radisson was not strong enough to do that but her toes on her front feet were moving slightly giving the impression she was trying to do that reflex. This was a very encouraging sign.

I told the party that I would stay for awhile with Radisson and suggested that they return home. One of the neighbors drove the Mapes' car home and the others followed in their own cars. Marna had decided to put on a pot of coffee earlier for the clients and there was still some left so we sat down and indulged in a cup. Marna volunteered to help clean up but I needed to stay for awhile and keep Radisson under observation, so I suggested she go home and be with the boys.

I cleaned the instruments and put the pack into the autoclave [machine that sterilizes surgical instruments using high-pressure steam]. It took almost an hour to return the hospital to its spic and span condition. During this time I checked on my patient every ten minutes. I brought a comfortable chair in from the reception room, poured the last cup of coffee from the pot, and sat down in front of Radisson's cage. The bell on the autoclave rang and I vented the machine. I entered all of the surgical data on the patient record. Antibiotics were injected into the muscle. Radisson was perking up. Her eyes were no longer glazed and she would visually follow me when I walked by her cage. She would even retract her foot slightly when I pinched her toe. The drip was slowed down to two drops per minute. It was a little past two in the morning when I locked up the premises and headed for home.

# 3 –

# ST. PATRICK'S CAT

**I** had my coat on and was just getting ready to leave my own hospital at day's end. Jo, my receptionist, flagged me down and wanted to go over a couple of cases that had scheduled appointments for the next day. The phone rang. The Hawthorne exchange was on the line and they were glad to have located me before I had left. A client with an injured cat was already on her way to the Hawthorne hospital. Could I meet them at that hospital? I replied that I would take the case and headed my Mustang north rather than east toward home.

I had asked Jo to call Marna and tell her to go ahead and have dinner and I would eat later. I arrived after the client. I unlocked the hospital and Mrs. Conway entered with her green and white cat. I took special note since I had never seen a cat of that color before. I located the client/patient card from the files. The cat's name was Star. She was a domestic short hair, white in color, female, and three years old. I invited Star and Mrs. Conway into the exam room.

Star had both patches and streaks of green paint on her. Mr. Conway had been painting some trim on their house when Star got the idea of jumping up on the stool beside him. The paint bucket and lid were there first. Star hit the edge of the lid that was partially hanging over the edge of the stool and it flipped over on top of her. That explained the green and white color. Star hit the ground on the run and proceeded to find protection for herself under the car. This provided a

12

good location for her to clean herself up. She now groomed herself by attempting to lick that terrible green stuff off—now paint decorated her face as well.

Besides being decorated for St. Patrick's Day, she was vomiting because she had ingested too much of the paint. I asked the owner if it was oil or water base. She did not know so I had her call home and find out from her husband. His answer was water base. That was good!

I put on a kennel smock and took Star to the grooming room and secured her to the tub. I directed Mrs. Conway to wait in the reception room. Much of the paint had dried in Star's fur. I gave Star a medicated bath and rinsed her down with as warm a water as I felt she would tolerate. Now she needed to be combed out. Most of the paint released its grip on the fur and collected on the teeth of the comb. I could wipe the comb on a paper towel and repeat the process. Finally Star looked almost completely white again. I then bathed her with Amway's LOC shampoo and that removed more of the green tinge. Star actually received three complete baths and when I toweled her down for the last time, there was even a green tint left on the towel.

Star had vomited enough so that no emetic was necessary but I gave her some Mylanta to coat her stomach to prevent any more after effects. I carried her out to Mrs. Conway and put her into her cage since all of the green paint that had rubbed off onto the cage was now dry. Mrs. Conway paid her bill and remarked that that was the most expensive bath Star would ever receive. The clean-up job took a little longer than usual. I put the towels that I had used to dry her off into the washing machine in hope that all of the green tint would wash out.

I called home to tell Marna I was on my way. When I entered our kitchen Marna had my dinner ready. She placed a glass of ice tea in front of me and then sat down while I ate and brought me up to the minute on the day's events. As I was finishing, the boys came into the house and wanted to share with me some of their school papers that had been returned. Before I had completed my perusal of their homework the phone rang.

San Pedro had a party on the line with a kitten that had been mangled by the aggressive neighborhood tomcat. I changed into more comfortable clothes and was on my way again.

The kitten was brought into the hospital in a cardboard cat carrier. It was crying loudly all of the time. The Dunkins asked me to put the kitten to sleep. They had the kitten for only a week and had not become too attached to it in that short period of time. I suggested a cursory exam before a final decision was made.

The kitten that they had named Ned was in bad shape. This long-hair feline was about six weeks in age and yellow in color. A huge patch of skin was missing under the neck and many puncture wounds were evident on it's shoulder and neck. Mr. Dunkin said if it was going to cost over fifty dollars, to put the animal to sleep. I explained that thirty-five dollars was already invested and that it would cost another twenty to euthanize the kitten. He said, "Go ahead and put it out of its misery."

It was a hard thing to do but I agreed with him. The kitten would require considerable surgery and at that point I did not know how much internal damage might have occurred. This assurance made them feel better. The necessary documents were signed, the charges tendered, and the clients departed. I took care of the grim task before me and headed for home.

It was past midnight when the phone rang. I was connected to the client through the Gardena exchange switchboard. Mr. Boswell had a Doberman named Charger that had gotten into a fight. Some of his bite wounds would probably require suturing. I agreed to meet him at that location in a half hour.

I washed my face, dressed, and headed northeast in my Mustang. Mr. Boswell pulled into the parking lot at the same time. Charger was tied in the back of Mr. Boswell's pick-up truck. He growled at me as I got out of my car. I heeded the warning and asked Mr. Boswell to follow me into the hospital. He untied Charger and soon both had joined me.

He lifted his seventy-pound plus dog up on the exam table and I made a cursory exam of the lacerations. I decided it would be best to do the suturing in the treatment room so he lifted Charger down and followed me to the rear of the hospital. This time he patted the top of the table and told Charger to jump up. The Doberman was instantly on the table where I could perform the necessary surgery.

Charger insisted on facing me at all times so I requested Mr. Boswell to hold his pet's neck to one side. Under the surgery light many old scars were evident as well as two fresh gashes that would require my atten-tion. I got out a syringe full of intravenous anesthetic and prepared to administer it. I then asked Mr. Boswell to hold Charger's leg so that I could locate a vein.

"He don't need that stuff in his vein!" was Mr. Boswell's immediate reply.

"Those wounds will require suturing," I replied.

"Put some of that other stuff around the cuts!"

"I can't use what is in the syringe. I will have to use a different type of anesthetic."

While I was filling another syringe with xylocaine, we carried on a continuous conversation.

"Are you sure you can hold him still for me?" I asked.

"Doc, look at all those scars. All were fixed while he was a-standing and me a-holding him."

"Okay, I'll try, but hold him firmly."

"Will do!"

Charger stood there motionless while I first blocked the injured areas and then sutured them. Mr. Boswell thanked me for doing the surgery as he had directed. He snapped his fingers and pointed to the floor. Charger jumped down.

We returned to the front desk to settle the account. He suggested that it would be a good idea to put his dog in the truck before it made a mess on the floor. I said, "That sounds like a good idea to me. Go ahead!" A moment later I looked up and his white beat-up pick-up with a rusty colored tailgate was pulling out of the parking lot. I was upset because he had not paid his bill. My contract for emergencies included the emergency fee and half of any anesthetic and X rays that were provided. I had just done surgery for nothing!

The address he gave me was not far away so I waited about ten minutes and phoned him. An operator came on the line and said, "This number is no longer in service." I was really upset now. It was late and I thought it would be best to go to his house in the morning to collect my fee.

I got back home in time to get some sleep. I got up early and indulged in a quick breakfast then headed for the Gardena area. With my Thomas Guide on my lap and a slip of paper with the Boswell address in hand I looked for the residence in question. The address turned out to be a vacant lot. I had been taken!

# 4 -

# HOT FEET

**I** have learned one thing for certain—it impossible to schedule emergencies. If I attempt to anticipate one by waiting, no emergency occurs. If I am busy doing something important, the phone rings. Emergencies can occur any day of the week and any time of day. They rarely fit into my schedule, but life is full of the unexpected.

I had not commenced any complicated chores around the house Saturday afternoon because I am usually very involved treating emergency cases. No calls came in all afternoon. Since I was home, the boys urged me to barbecue. I started the fire and waited for the phone to ring. It didn't. I placed the chicken on the grill and the phone still did not ring. I turned the chicken the first time and finally the phone rang. Marna came outside and informed me that the Palos Verdes exchange was on the line. Marna is my personal switchboard operator. She receives calls from the four answering services which in turn do business with the twelve hospitals for which I take emergencies. The operator cross-connected me to the client. Their Dalmatian had burnt its front feet.

I met the Walters at the Palos Verdes hospital. Their dog, Comet, a four-year-old female, had to be carried in. The pads on her front feet were painful and she was reluctant to walk on them. In the examination room I was able to perform a more definitive exam. Comet's feet had lineal burns on them like she had stepped on a floor furnace grate. Mr. Walters said that he had been barbecuing and Comet had tried to steal the meat off the grill.

16

"She had taken some chicken off about two weeks ago and gotten away with it. I do start my chicken on a cold grill but today I was cooking ribs and they were almost done. The grill was very hot. I went into the house for a moment and left the barbecue unattended never thinking Comet would grab anything from a hot grill. I heard her yelp from the kitchen and when I went out, she was on the lawn licking her feet. One side of ribs was askew on the grill. This was evidence that she had tried to grab them but quit when she burnt her feet. I tried to check her paws but she was too busy licking them to allow me to investigate."

I checked Comet's feet. They were burnt but probably more pain was caused than injury. A protective layer of furacin ointment was applied. Since she was still trying to lick her feet, she needed to have them band-aged. Some roller gauze was first applied and then elastic tape completed the task. Burn lesions were noticed on her muzzle, but I felt they would heal without treatment. No ointment would last very long anyway in that location. Mr. Walter lifted Comet from the exam table and placed her on the floor. She gave us a woeful look and just stood there. Now she didn't want to walk on her bandaged feet.

Mrs. Walters took care of the account and her husband carried Comet out to their car. I led the way and opened the back of the station wagon. I told Mr. Walters that if she chewed off the bandages in the next day or two that it would be okay to just let the feet heal without additional protection. The Walters apologized for disturbing me that afternoon and said, "I hope that Comet learned a lesson. Time will tell if she needs to be watched more carefully in the future."

I returned home to find that Allen had completed the chicken and done a superb job of it. Marna had prepared a tossed green salad. Allen had even toasted a loaf of garlic bread on the barbecue and did not burn it as I frequently do. My family had been waiting for me to return. We sat outside on the patio while Greta exercised her neck watching each one of us indulge in the chicken. We never allow her to be in any eating area so she stationed herself about fifteen feet away on the lawn. She monitored us very carefully. Greta started to get up and come over when Albert dropped a bone, but a stern command from me indicated to her that it was best to remain where she was.

I was up and on my way early Sunday morning for I had to visit five hospitals for morning treatments. I had mentally arranged my stops in a fashion so that when I got to the larger hospitals, I would be there when the morning kennel staff was there to assist me. This would speed me up a good bit for this extra assistance was invaluable.

I backed the Mustang out of the garage and was just getting ready to drive away when I noticed Marna frantically waving at me from the back door. The answering service was on the line. The call involved a cat with a swollen shoulder. I decided to change my preplanned routing and go there first even though it was one of my later scheduled stops. After all, animals in immediate need require my attention first.

It was going to take the Kramers thirty minutes to get to the hospital with their cat Felicia. With this delay in mind, I decided to drive west to the coast and then take the scenic ride south along the Pacific Ocean to my destination. As I approached Redondo Beach the smell of salt air permeated the car. I rolled my window down even further to absorb the fresh air. There were wisps of fog rising off the ocean only to disappear as the morning sun evaporated them. It was a pleasant trip south with very little traffic on an early Sunday morning.

I was even able to get all of my cases treated before the Kramers arrived with Felicia. I had already pulled the client/patient card from the files so we went to the treatment room where I could inspect the swollen shoulder. A soft swelling existed over her right scapula and her temperature was well above normal. Two small puncture wounds were also noted and these three things combined were pathognomonic for an abscess. The swollen shoulder had bothered Felicia considerably for there were numerous abrasions present caused by claws of her back foot.

Mrs. Kramer held Felicia while I injected some surital into the vein on her front leg. The Kramers returned to the reception room. I lanced the abscess which turned out to be quite large. Considerable purulent matter exuded from the infected area. An antiseptic solution was used to lavage the area and forte, an antibiotic ointment, was applied into the abscessed area. Next a seton drain was established to enable the area to stay open so it could be medicated for several days. I gave my patient an injection of penicillin in the muscle and then caged her in the recovery ward.

The Kramers were brought up to date regarding the surgery and aftercare. They wanted to take Felicia home. I escorted them to the back of the hospital. When they saw their cat and smelled the putrid odor of the drained abscess, they changed their minds. I never even had the opportunity to discourage them about releasing their pet at this time. They even recommended that they pick up Felicia on their way home from work on Monday. I said that this would be great, since the hospital staff could give Felicia a medicated bath to remove the stench from her coat. They left the customary deposit and said they would call in the morning to see how their cat was doing.

I then cleaned up, rechecked Felicia, and headed for the door. I had two cases that required a recheck at Lawndale and then proceeded to Hawthorne for my third stop of the morning. I had to retape an ear on a Schnauzer pup that had had its ears cropped. When I finished treating that wiggling exuberant pup, I had to readjust the splint on a fracture case and add a bit more tape in the places where the patient had been chewing. A hospitalized Shelty was lonesome and now whined as I closed the ward door.

When I got to Manhattan Beach the kennel staff asked that I call home. Marna had a call from the Torrance hospital. I quickly finished treating the Manhattan Beach cases. The staff would get the pets that needed my attention and bring them into the treatment room. One of the staff would hold the pet while I rendered whatever medical attention was necessary and then it was returned to a clean cage that had been prepared by another member of the staff while it had been vacated.

I took a detour in my planned treatment schedule again and went to the Torrance hospital. Mr. Beverly was waiting in his car with Tongo, a mixture of what appeared to be a Border Collie and who knows what else. Tongo had a six inch gaping wound on his chest. Mr. Beverly had no idea how or where it had happened. When he fed Tongo that morning he noticed the bleeding wound.

The area to be sutured was near Tongo's head and would require him to be anesthetized. I used a short-acting anesthetic and did the suturing while he was relaxed and under my control rather than taking a risk of being bitten.

When surgery was completed, Mr. Beverly took care of the charges and we went to the recovery ward to get Tongo. He was waking up and, unfortunately, had vomited his breakfast then rolled in it. Mr. Beverly looked at me with a "what to do" glance and I suggested that a clean-up bath would be appropriate. Tongo was rather unsteady on his feet, so his owner held him upright in the tub while I gave him a bath.

Tongo was rinsed off, I toweled him down, then we put him into the cage dryer for a few minutes. Soon he was sufficiently dry to send home. I reminded Mr. Beverly to call in the morning and make two appointments—one in three days for a recheck and one in two weeks for suture removal.

By the time I had arrived at the next scheduled location that Sunday morning, all of the staff had completed their jobs and departed. Fortunately only three animals required my care and soon I was heading for Palos Verdes for my final morning treatment. It was almost noon and well past church service time, so my coat and tie that had occupied the back seat all morning would be unused that particular day.

When I pulled into the hospital parking lot, two clients were waiting. One had been there for over half an hour. Marna had told the exchange where I would be and the service had directed them to this hospital. The second client had arrived unexpectedly. The clients had occupied their time by visiting with each other.

The scheduled appointment was seen first. Miss Conklin had Minnie in her arms. I filled out the medical record card and recorded the anamnesis [history]. Minnie was a shorthaired, tortoise shell, spayed female cat. She had not been eating for two or three days. She belonged to a flight attendant who had been gone during that period of time. Minnie had not eaten any food from the automatic cat feeder—it was still full. Miss Conklin had left on flights before and left Minnie locked in the house with ample food, water, and a litter box and returned to find her cat was doing well. This was not the case when she returned this morning.

We went into the exam room and Miss Conklin placed Minnie on the table. Minnie's temperature was normal. No ingesta could be found in her bowels or her stomach. I was puzzled! I gave her a couple of droppers of a vitamin syrup that often stimulates the appetite. I then opened a can of cat food and offered it to her. She readily accepted it and started eating it ravenously. Miss Conklin and I got our heads together in an attempt to resolve the problem. I asked her to take me step by step through Minnie's eating habits. She said, "When I left early Friday morning, I added enough dry food to the automatic feeder to fill it up. I put out fresh water and cleaned the litter box. I do this every time I have to leave on a flight." I asked her to describe the automatic feeder. "It is one of those that you added food at the top and the little pellets come out the bottom as she eats." I suggested that when she got home to throw all of the food in the feeder out. Clean out the feeder, dry it well, and then put fresh food in it. I sent Miss Conklin and her cat home with some of the vitamin syrup I had given Minnie earlier. I recorded her telephone number on a scrap of paper and told Miss Conklin I would call later in the day to see how Minnie was doing.

The Wells came in next. They had picked up a puppy the week before from the humane society. The pup's name was Chardonnay. The little pup had Yorkshire Terrier blood in his veins but did not appear to be a pure-breed. He was vomiting, had diarrhea, and refused to eat. He was probably six to eight weeks old and as cute as a button. Mrs. Wells handed me a coupon from the pound entitling them to a courtesy health examination at any of the participating veterinary hospitals. At the bottom of the coupon in bold print was the statement: Good for free examination within 48 hours of purchase only. I pointed out this condition and read it to them for emphasis. The Wells said they were too busy to come in during the speci-fied time and even though the coupon had expired, they wondered if I would honor it. I explained that it was very important to have had their pup examined in that specific period of time. If the pup was unhealthy, it could have been returned to the pound and another pup selected. If it was healthy, then its vaccination program could be initiated.

I checked the pup over and was almost certain that the pup was infected with parvovirus. The only way I could be positive was to take some samples and send them to the laboratory for confirmation. I expressed to them that it was probably too late to change the course of the possible viral infection.

They asked what they owed me for they assumed that I would not accept the coupon. I told them there was no charge except for the labo-ratory expense if they desired to take that route. With tears in their eyes they picked Chardonnay up. They thanked me and headed for the door after remarking, "We'll return him to the pound and will start off properly the next time." I thoroughly sterilized the table in the exam room and was thankful that they had held Chardonnay in their arms while he was in the hospital.

I decided to call Miss Conklin since Minnie was still on my mind. She had cleaned out the feeder as directed. "When I emptied the plastic feeder, some of the pellets stuck to the side. I looked at it carefully and noticed a fine mildew or mold. I took some fresh pellets from the bag and scattered them on the floor. Minnie was interested immediately. Her food must have either tasted bad or smelled bad or both. She was wise not to consume any of the food or I may have been there [hospital] for other reasons." She thanked me for the return call and promised to be more careful in feeding Minnie in the future. I reminded her to be certain the feeder was absolutely dry before she refilled it.

I arrived home a little after three in the afternoon. I was ready for a nap but the boys wanted me to join them in the backyard. They wanted to play catch but I begged off. I told them that I would watch. I settled into a lounge chair and did watch for awhile before I fell asleep. Marna came out to visit me and Albert told her that I was watching them play, but my eyes were closed. I woke up when George shook me by the shoulder and handed me a glass of iced tea. Allen had started the barbecue and I was delegated to watch him—with my eyes open. I marveled at how each of my sons had anticipated my needs.

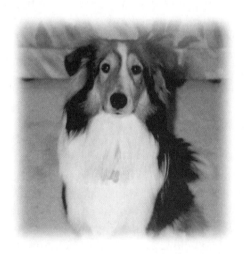

# 5

# TWO HAPPY BOYS

Jo and I were watching Mrs. Milton walking down the sidewalk toward my hospital. Tasha, a Samoyed, always walks as far away from the traffic as possible until she approaches my hospital. Then she would cross over to the other side of her handler to get as far away as possible from our premises. The walk was a routine affair and we were able to witness the event daily except during inclement weather.

It would make no difference whether they passed going east or west, the crossover event would happen. When Tasha was a safe distance from my hospital, she would maneuver to again be as far away from the passing traffic as possible. Sometimes clients would watch this maneuver with us. Jo would say, "Now," and within a step or two Tasha would move to the outside. Tasha had made numerous visits to the hospital for variable reasons and was showing her disdain for us by her actions. It became a topic of conversation whenever the Miltons brought Tasha into the hospital. It also made no difference which member of the family escorted Tasha down the street. Mom, Dad, Carey, or Robert—all got the same result. We got to know the Miltons quite well for they lived only a couple of blocks away.

I had just completed a late surgery and Jo had graciously consented to stay and help me clean up the hospital to prepare for the morning appointments. When the premise was spic and span we headed for the parking lot. Jo was backing out her car and I was locking the front door when both Carey and Robert appeared on the scene. In their hands they held a box that contained a rabbit. The boys' rabbit, Ears, was not doing well and had lost a lot of weight. Their father had told them that if Ears was not better in a couple of day, Ears should be put to sleep. Two teary eyed youngsters about eight and ten looked up at me. They were broken hearted for Ears was a special friend of theirs.

Jo saw me looking into the box and returned to see if I needed any assistance. All four of us went into the examination room. The boys' father had phoned the boys and told them to bring Ears down that afternoon for euthanasia, but the boys had procrastinated and waited until the last minute to make that final decision.

Carey, the older of the two boys, took on the roll of spokesman. "Daddy said to put Ears to sleep."

"Let me take a look at him first, Carey."

"Okay."

"How long has Ears been like this?"

Carey looked at his brother, Robert. Robert only shrugged his shoulders. Finally they agreed on a time. Carey said, "When vacation started."

"When was school over?" I inquired.

"Last month."

"Let's see, that would be about five weeks wouldn't it?"

"Yeah," responded Robert.

Ears was very emaciated and his temperature was below normal. He was well groomed and cared for otherwise. Upon further questioning of the boys, I learned that Ears was hardly eating anything even though he spent a good deal of time at his feeding dish because the food was always scattered around his cage. This indicated to me that Ears was hungry but for some reason was unable to eat. With this information in mind I had Jo hold Ears and I opened his mouth. Ear's incisor teeth had grown to such a degree that he was unable to close his mouth completely let alone be able to chew anything that he could get into his mouth.

"When are you going to do it, doctor?"

I looked up at Jo and tears were welling up in her eyes. "Let me try something first. Will that be alright with you, boys?"

"Yeah," they said in unison.

I asked them to go out to the reception room for a few minutes while Jo and I took Ears to the treatment room. Jo held Ears securely while I trimmed his four front teeth with a dental instrument. About an inch of each tooth now lay on the treatment table. My greatest concern was the possibility that Ears had progressed past the point of likely recovery. I wanted to give my patient some life support energy so I administered sixty milliliters of 5 percent saline and dextrose under his skin at the back of his neck. Ears never objected at all as he was so weak. Jo put him into a temporary cage and I returned to the front desk.

"Is he dead yet?" asked Robert.

"No!" I responded, "I think there is a chance for him to be well again."

"Daddy said to put him to sleep," said Robert.

I explained to the boys that Ears was starving to death.

"He had plenty of food," said Carey.

"Ears couldn't eat it, Carey."

"Why?"

"His teeth are too long."

"Can we see him?" asked Robert.

Jo brought Ears out to the exam room. I gave the boys instructions about caring for Ears and then asked them to bring their rabbit back on Monday morning for me to see again. The boys left the hospital. Carey was holding the box that contained Ears. Robert and Carey were all smiles. Robert nudged his brother when they exited the door and said, "Maybe Ears will live, won't he, Carey?" Jo and I watched the boys walk down the sidewalk. Two young boys had entered the hospital with long faces and tears running down their cheeks. Now they were leaving with dry eyes and smiles. We smiled and felt good too.

Monday morning came and Mr. Milton arrived a few minutes after the hospital opened. He said, "I gave the boys money to pay for putting Ears to sleep but they returned with both the rabbit and the money. They told me what you had done and I want to thank you. Ears is eating! He is showing signs of improvement and getting lots of attention from Carey and Robert. It certainly was a happy household when I got home from work on Saturday. I was concerned that the decision to put Ears to sleep had only been delayed. I really think that he is going to survive."

We chatted awhile about both Tasha and Ears. Finally he said, "I came in to settle my account." I told him that I had already been paid in full for my services. My payment was seeing two happy boys walk out of the door. He still insisted, but I politely refused.

On Monday I saw Ears again. He was doing well and hopping around in a limited fashion. Each of the boys tried to outtalk the other as they attempted to bring me up to date since I had seen them last. Friday morning Carey and Robert brought Ears down to the hospital to show me how much Ears had improved. Robert was carrying a small box.

"These cookies are for you," blurted Robert.

"Shh, they are supposed to be a surprise," said Carey.

Robert couldn't be contained for he added, "Carey and I decorated them after mother baked them."

A few weeks later when Mrs. Milton was walking Tasha and saw Jo and myself looking out the window, she came into the hospital dragging Tasha behind her. "Ears is doing fine now and I want to thank you." I suggested that she have the boys bring Ears in every other month and have me recheck his teeth. I explained that rabbits' teeth grow continuously and if they do not have anything hard to chew on like those in the wild, their teeth are not ground down properly. That is the reason Ears's teeth may have to be trimmed regularly. Jo and I thanked her for the delicious cookies that we enjoyed before she followed Tasha out the door.

I was on my way home from work that evening. As I was driving by a colleague's hospital, I noticed a beat-up white pickup with a rusty tailgate in his parking lot. I drove around the block and pulled in and parked right next to the pickup. I went in to talk to the doctor. The receptionist knew me and I asked if a Mr. Boswell was here with his Doberman named Charger. She said, "No," but a Mr. Williams was here with a Doberman named Charger. I quickly explained the reason I had stopped and asked her to see if Dr. Andrew could talk with me for a moment. He did.

I explained to Jack the experience I had had with a Mr. Boswell and thought he was now going by the name of Williams. He asked me to wait in his office and then asked his receptionist to phone the number that Mr. Williams had given them. It was no longer in service. The address on the client card was the same he had given me—a vacant lot.

Jack had been suturing Charger's lesions just as I had done. When he had completed his task, he made some excuse to put Charger into a run so he could relieve himself. He then confronted his client. "I had my receptionist phone your house. Your phone has been disconnected."

"I couldn't pay my last bill," was the response.

Jack repeated the address on the patient card and the client confirmed that it was correct. Jack said, "I know it is a vacant lot."

"Get me my dog."

The client was beginning to become very uneasy. Jack continued, "Is your name Boswell or Williams?"

"Get me my dog," he repeated.

He started shouting and was very upset. He followed Jack out to the front desk. Then he saw me standing there with a telephone to my ear. I was holding the phone and pretending to be talking to the Gardena police department. When he realized the situation he was facing, he asked the receptionist how much his bill was. He paid her that amount in cash. The he turned to me and paid his account with me in full with cash. The kennel person brought Charger up and Mr. Boswell or Mr. Williams left in a hurry. We never did find out what his real name was. Jack said he owed me a lunch. I said that I owed Jack a lunch since he had helped me to collect a bad debt. We resolved the situation by alternately taking each other out to lunch.

I had a late emergency trip to make that evening. When I got home the boys were asleep but Greta wasn't. She was in our bedroom trying to get under our bed. She whined as she tried to get under the bed on one side and then would run around to the other side and repeat her actions. I decided to take a look for myself. I located a flashlight and looked under the bed. Several boxes were stored there in an area that was barely six inches high. I pulled a couple of boxes out and Greta sniffed them thoroughly and then returned to her previous antics. One more box was removed to provide me with a more complete view. Reflected in the beam of the flashlight were two big yellow eyes. We had an uninvited visitor that had staked out a claim under our bed. A few weeks before, I had installed a cat entry door in the back door. Faux Pas, our Siamese cat, could now come and go. Our feline stranger had taken advantage of this newly installed entrance to gain access to our abode.

The boys were asleep so we quietly shut their bedroom doors. Faux Pas was located and put into one of the boy's rooms. All of the rest of the doors in the house were closed leaving only a passageway down the hall, across the kitchen, and through the utility room to the great outdoors. We left Greta in to chase the cat out the door.

I lifted up the foot of the bed. Marna used a broom to make a few passes under the bed before "big yellow eyes" beat a hasty retreat. The only place the stranger could exit was via the path we had established to the back door. The cat had no time to investigate any other hiding places because Greta was just a leap or two behind. Our guest exited as planned and disappeared into the night. I secured the cat portal on the door so that Faux Pas or her friends would be unable to use it. The boxes were put back under the bed and Marna let Faux Pas out of the boys' bedroom. We looked at each other and laughed. The boys had missed all of the excitement involving the mysterious visitor and the big chase.

At breakfast the following morning, I related the previous night's experience to my three disbelieving sons. I got the broom and escorted the boys to our bedroom and re-enacted the event. Greta was the most attentive and was a perfect character actor for the great chase—she performed well trying to get under the bed and then when I shouted, "There goes the cat!" she chased an invisible cat through the same exit route as the night before. I left for the office after measuring for a new back door. On the way home that night I stopped at the lumber company and brought home the new door to install. I thought the cat door was a good idea but I was proven wrong.

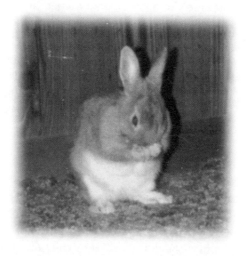

# 6

## Big Green Eyes

**I**t was about two in the morning when the phone rang. I reached for the receiver and knocked the phone off my nightstand. I had to turn on the light and scramble for the phone before I awakened the entire family. The Hawthorne service was on the line and they patched me to the client, Mrs. Quigley, who had an emergency problem with Nikki.

Nikki was having trouble breathing and was making strange sounds when he inhaled or exhaled. According to his owner, he would stand with his head held low and his neck stretched like it was a real effort to breathe. It sounded like a bona fide emergency so I agreed to meet her at the Torrance hospital immediately. I was out of the house within five minutes and on my way.

I arrived first and Mrs. Quigley a few minutes later. She carried Nikki, a male standard poodle, because she felt that a leash was inappropriate to use considering his stressful condition. Nikki was in deep trouble. He was in severe respiratory distress. An abraded area on his neck was noted and upon palpation of his throat, it became apparent that several laryngeal cartilages were damaged. I had Mrs. Quigley hold Nikki while I went to the Mustang for the anesthetic machine and then a short acting anesthetic was given intravenously.

The neck area was trimmed and an incision was made over the partially collapsed trachea. Muscles were parted and the trachea exposed. I was now able to proceed with a tracheotomy. As soon as the trachea was opened slightly, Nikki took a deep breath of fresh air. The wheezing noise of his attempted inhalation immediately ceased. I inserted an adapter that fit into his trachea and attached it to the oxygen on the machine. Nikki was now getting plenty of oxygen and his breathing was normal. I disconnected the oxygen supply and allowed Nikki to breathe on his own through the adapter. He was now doing fine. The adapter was securely taped into the proper position so he could not misplace it when he fully recovered from the anesthetic. I now caged Nikki and went out to talk to Mrs. Quigley to find out more about this unusual case.

Nikki had been chained in the back yard because he wanted to jump the fence and visit his lady friend down the street. He had been given a twenty-five foot radius to roam in and the chain was anchored in the middle of the lawn. He had access to his water dish, food pan, doghouse, and his favorite lounging area by the backdoor.

The Quigleys had misjudged the length of the chain and Nikki had jumped over the fence on his way to have an affair with his female friend. The chain was long enough for him to clear the fence, but not long enough for him to place all four of his feet on the ground. Only his back feet could touch mother earth. He was getting tired of standing on his back feet with his front feet on the fence and was gradually choking to death.

Mrs. Quigley had awakened when she heard him scratching somewhere and went out in the backyard to investigate. She observed the chain disappearing over the fence. She said, "I quickly went through the house to the front yard and there was my Nikki with his back feet on the ground, his tongue out of his mouth, and his eyes bulging. I lifted him off the ground but couldn't release the chain that was now slack. Somehow I managed to push him back over the fence. Then I returned through the house to render whatever first aid I could. I pumped his chest to help him breathe. He was breathing some because I could hear that terrible sound. I then called you. I loaded Nikki into the car seat beside me. Once when he did not make any sounds for a bit, I pulled over to feel his chest. I could feel his heart beating so I pumped his chest again."

We went into the critical care ward and looked at Nikki. He was trying to raise his head in response to his owner's voice. I said that I would wait awhile and keep an eye on Nikki. Mrs. Quigley wanted to stay also, so I asked her to put on a pot of coffee for us while I cleaned up the instruments and returned the treatment room to normal. Mrs. Quigley had done an amazing job and had gotten Nikki to me in the nick of time. The poodle's neck was badly bruised and swollen by now due to both his trauma and to surgery. We checked on Nikki one more time. He was wobbly but on his feet and watching us through the cage door. We decided it was time to leave. I had appointments that started early and a couple of surgeries on my morning's docket.

When I pulled away from the hospital, the rays of the morning sun were just visible in the east as they crept over the San Bernadino Mountains. I was able to indulge in a short catnap in my leather chair before shaving. Then a quick breakfast with Marna and I was on my way for a day at my hospital.

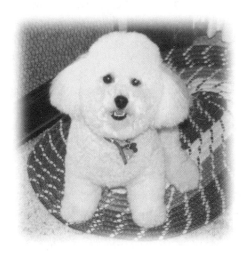

# 7

# A RECOUNT

**S**unday had rolled around again and I had only one hospital other than my own that had pets to check. I was up early and treated several animals at the Hawthorne hospital. Soon I was on my way home to attend church with my family. Marna had the boys ready and we, as usual, played follow the leader as we drove to church in our separate cars. George accompanied me to church because his two brothers wanted to ride with me on the way home.

Before I left home, I called the different answering services to give them my game plan for the morning. I was going to church first, my hospital next, and then home. The boys attended Sunday School while Marna and I listened to a very inspirational sermon. I was able to hear the entire sermon as the ushers did not have to interrupt me by calling me to the phone in the narthex.

Allen and Albert joined me in the Mustang as I headed for Redondo Beach. I was glad to have the extra help that morning since my kennel staff had requested the weekend off. As I pulled into the parking lot, I could hear the telephone ringing. It was still ringing persistently as I unlocked the front door. The Manhattan Beach operator was on the line. I was greeted with, "Doctor, you have been hard to locate. I called your church and the service was over, I called your hospital and no answer, no one was at your residence so I called your hospital again. I figured that you were in transit. Can you take this call

32

about a dog trying to give birth?" I was patched through to Mrs. Wingate who had a German Shepherd named Tammy who was in whelp but was having difficulty. "I do not know how to assist my dog. She is as big as a blimp and must have at least a dozen pups wanting to come into this world of ours." I informed her that I was about thirty minutes away from the Manhattan Beach hospital and asked Mrs. Wingate to meet me there.

While I was on the phone, Allen had already taken charge of cleaning the nine cages that were occupied. He showed his younger brother, Albert, the proper way to clean cages and handle the occupants. Allen brought the two patients that needed my morning attention into the treatment room while Allen's assistant, Albert, cleaned their cages. Soon all the chores were done and the three of us were on our way north to Manhattan Beach.

We arrived first and Allen and I located what we thought might be needed to deliver the pups. Albert waited out front for the client to arrive. I looked for the client/patient card but could not locate one. Apparently this was a new client for this hospital.

Albert showed Mrs. Wingate and her daughter, Karen, into the treatment room. Tammy followed them on a leash. I was informed that no pups had arrived as yet. "If they don't arrive soon, I fear that she will burst." I agreed with her after I had a good look at Tammy. Allen and I lifted Tammy up on the treatment table. She started straining again. I gloved and digitally checked the birth canal. I could feel the nose of a fetus and it appeared to be in the proper position to come into the world. Tammy must have broken water some time ago for the birth canal was dry. Mrs. Wingate decided to retreat to the reception room with her daughter. I located a substitute lubrication preparation and applied it to the birth canal. Next I gave Tammy an injection of the hormone oxytocin to enable her to continue her strong contractions.

That was all that was needed to put whelping into motion. The first pup was dead but the rest started arriving faster than I could handle them by myself. I would open the amniotic sack and clamp off the umbilical cord. Allen would get them breathing and hand them to Albert to dry off. Albert would then put the new arrivals into a box that Allen had previously prepared. Allen was instructing his brother in a very professional manner and the entire event went very smoothly.

Soon the box was full of squirming noisy pups. Tammy was very interested in joining them. I followed with another lighter dose of the hormone so she could expel any afterbirth. Tammy and her progeny were then put into a large cage so the young pups could nurse.

I asked my sons to count the pups—Allen counted ten and Albert only nine. We rechecked the count together and finally agreed that Allen's count had been correct.

Albert went out front and invited Mrs. Wingate and her daughter to come back and visit the new family. Albert was very excited and started telling Karen, who was about his age, all about his part in the birthing of the pups. We counted all of the pups again and all five of us agreed that ten was the correct number. The pups were put back into the box and Allen carried it out to the reception room. When he returned we lifted Tammy into the tub to wash off her rear quarters. I proceeded to clean up the treatment room while Allen did the bathing. Suddenly Allen said, "Tammy's straining again!" I assumed that he meant that the afterbirth was being discharged but he informed me, "Here comes another pup!" He brought the newborn to me and I clamped off its umbilicus and then tied it off with suture material as I had done to the others. Now we had eleven live pups. Tammy had delivered a full dozen.

I asked Allen to go out front and bring the box of pups back to me. "Don't say a word about the last pup." All three of us went out in front with the box full of German Shepherd pups. I asked Karen to count the pups again for sometimes my sons do not count correctly. I winked at Mrs. Wingate as Karen did the recount. Karen said, "I think there are eleven but they are so wiggly that I may have counted one twice." She counted them two more times and each count indicated that she had been correct the first time. I then told her that I had added another one to the box in the back room. Allen carried the box of eleven out to the Wingate camper and Albert led Tammy. Soon the boys were back helping me complete the task of cleaning up before we headed home.

We arrived home and had to explain to Marna why we were so late. I had neglected to call her when I changed locations, and she had no idea where she could locate us. That was a definite oversight on my part.

# 8

# THE STALKER

I was on my way to Lawndale to respond to a case involving an aged dog. The owners, the Wilcoxes, had mentioned that Bitsy, their sixteen-year-old poodle, may be hanging on to her last threads of life. I reached my destination in about twenty minutes and that gave me time to remove my gas anesthetic machine from the trunk of my Mustang and assemble it in case the use of oxygen gas was necessary. As I rolled the machine into the hospital, the Wilcoxes arrived.

In Mr. Wilcox's arms was Bitsy. Bitsy was old. His silver color blended into the grayness of age, which did give him the appearance of a much younger dog, but his physical appearance belayed that assumption. Bitsy was placed on a blanket so he would not be exposed to the cold stainless steel table. The dog's head would rise when anyone spoke or moved but soon he would rest it on the blanket giving all of us an indication he was about to give up his lease on life.

I placed my stethoscope on his chest. I detected an irregular heartbeat and his pulse was very weak. His color was not the usual pink, indicating that his oxygen supply was insufficient. I commenced by passing a tracheal tube down the dog's breathing passages but without the short acting anesthetic or sedative that I would usually use to accomplish this task in a more viable dog. Then I turned on the oxygen supply. His color improved markedly.

We watched him for some time and then I suggested that they go home for there was nothing they could do. Mr. Wilcox rolled the machine with the oxygen supply still attached into the critical care ward while I carried Bitsy. Mrs. Wilcox followed. Together we watched Bitsy for almost forty minutes as their dog seemed to be improving and resting well. I again suggested that they return home and I promised to stay with Bitsy for awhile. After they went out to their car, I locked the front door and picked up a chair from the reception room and headed for the critical care ward and my patient.

I had just entered the ward when Bitsy gave one deep inhalation followed by a prolonged expiration. I grabbed my stethoscope that was over my neck and listened. There was no sound. Bitsy's heart had stopped. I hurried to the front door and exited the hospital. I saw the Wilcox car still in the parking lot. They were in the front seat crying. I informed them of the circumstance. They had suspected that their beloved pet had only a few more hours to live. Mr. Wilcox said that he would come back into the hospital as soon as he composed himself. He took care of his account and asked me to make arrangements for the local pet cemetery to pick up Bitsy in the morning.

Mr. Wilcox said that Bitsy's passing was unusually hard for them. They had purchased Bitsy the same week their only son was born. Two months ago their son was killed in an automobile accident and from that time on Bitsy seemed to deteriorate more rapidly. "Thank you for all you have done, doctor." With that he left to join his wife in the car. I cleaned up the hospital and put Bitsy in a bag then headed for the front door. The Wilcox car was still in the parking lot. I put my anesthetic machine into the trunk of the Mustang and walked over to their car and asked them if I could be of any help. They weren't in any condition to drive anywhere, so I invited them to go across the street with me and have a cup of coffee.

We had a couple of cups of coffee each and just talked. Mrs. Wilcox said, "It is so hard to release a pet from life here on earth." I agreed and said that it is even more difficult to do that when the emotions of losing their pet is a reminder about the loss of their son. We chatted for awhile and then returned to our automobiles and went our separate ways. I gave a lot of thought about Bitsy and the Wilcoxes as I headed south toward home. I must have still been showing my emotions on my face when I entered my house, for Marna immediately asked me what was the matter.

Marna was enjoying a cup of coffee and brought me a cup in the family room. I was just beginning to relate the evening's experience to her when the phone rang. I had to make a return visit to Manhattan Beach to take care of an injured cat. I said goodnight to the boys and gave Marna a hug and a peck on the cheek and headed for the car. Marna followed me out with another cup of steaming coffee to enjoy on my trip. By this time I was completely saturated with coffee, and I knew that I would be able to keep my eyes open for a long time as I headed back up the coast.

The Williamsons were knocking on the door when I arrived. I unlocked the door and we went immediately into the exam room. They were clients of that hospital so I pulled the client/patient folder and returned to the examination room. In the meantime they had removed K. C. (Kitty Cat) from his cage and he was resting apprehensively in Mrs. Williamson's arms. She placed him on the table and I was looking at a twelve-year-old, black and white shorthaired, altered male cat. K. C. had an injured left front leg. He would not put any weight on it and objected when I gently attempted to rotate it. I suggested an X ray and the owners consented.

I returned fifteen minutes later with the wet radiograph and positioned it on the view screen. I was able to point out a fracture of the radius. The bone was not separated completely but there was a very evident spiral crack midshaft. I discussed the correction that was needed and felt that a splint would be a satisfactory way to protect and stabilize the leg so that it would have the opportunity to heal properly.

I brought in the anesthetic machine from the car. Mrs. Williamson held K. C. while I administered a short-acting anesthetic intravenously and then passed the appropriate size endotrachial tube and connected K. C. to the metafane gas. The Williamsons retired to the reception room and I carried K. C. into the treatment room dragging the anesthetic machine behind me. A feline size metasplint was fashioned to fit the leg properly. Next the splint was liberally padded with cotton and then the leg was firmly and securely taped to the splint so that any blood supply to the foot would not be impeded. The walking splint was now in place and the anesthetic machine was disconnected. K. C. was placed in a cage in the recovery ward.

I went to the front of the hospital to talk to the Williamsons and give them instructions concerning K. C.'s aftercare. I remarked that I had not noticed he was declawed until I positioned the metasplint. Mr. Williamson said that declawing K. C. was a must. "K. C.'s nickname is 'stalker.'" Mrs. Williamson said, "K. C. will stalk anything at any time. He will even stalk his food dish. He will place each foot gently down as he moves cautiously forward like he is walking on eggs. Just the tip of his tail will move. When he gets ready to pounce on the object, his tail will become motionless and then he crouches. His eyes become transfixed on the object of his attention. Then he will leap and grasp the object and in most cases just play with it."

"Kitty Cat will even stalk people and that is what got him into trouble this time. We had friends over for supper and put on a video of our trip to Norway. K. C. silently approached Mark who was holding a drink in his hand. All of us were watching television and were unaware of the cat's presence. All of a sudden there was a huge interruption. Mark gave a yell and flung his arms out. The glass and contents went everywhere. K. C. was thrown against the coffee table and quickly retired to the back of the house. He was noticeably limping as he made his exit. I brought him back out to the living room to show him the damage he had caused. He didn't want to place the left foot down and cried when we touched it. Mark and his wife felt really bad about K. C.'s injury. When the evening was over, they apologized again and headed for home. We were going to wait until tomorrow but decided that if we had an injury of this nature, we would want care immediately. That's why we called you."

I repeated the instructions for their cat's aftercare and asked them to call their regular veterinarian within twenty-four hours and give him a progress report and schedule an appointment for the splint removal. I took the anesthetic machine out to the car, disassembled it, and placed the parts in the styrofoam slots in the trunk of my car. I returned to the hospital, cleaned up the premises, and put everything away. Then I headed home. I checked with Marna this time to be certain that no other calls were pending.

The boys were sound asleep when I arrived. Marna had just made some coffee so we each had a cup and retired to the living room and sat on the couch. We enjoyed a cup of Starbucks' best and brought each other up on the day's events.

Albert came wandering out in a sleepy-eyed manner and crawled up on the couch between Marna and me. He snuggled in and was asleep again within ten minutes. Marna carefully got up and refilled our cups. We sat there quietly enjoying the peacefulness of the fireplace and finally gave up when the embers of the fire had faded. I picked Albert up and returned him to his bed and gave him a kiss as I pulled his blanket up and tucked him in.

# — 9 —

# AN INEBRIATED GOOSE

Salty edged his way into my practice in a very auspicious manner. He was presented to me by the Truffits with a "here he is" attitude and "please fix him up." Salty was plunked down on the exam table. At first glance I thought I was looking at a canine sumo wrestler. He was so pendulous in his abdominal area that it was difficult for him to stand. He preferred to sit on his rump and spin around facing the way that garnered his attention. It would have been much easier for me to examine him if he had been placed on a heavy-duty lazy Susan. Salty preferred to sit. In this position the weight of his abdominal area settled in the lower portion of his body enabling him to breath with less difficulty. This posture allowed the lungs to expand without competing with the diaphragmatic pressure against his thorax.

The Westie did not really walk at all—he waddled like an inebriated goose. When he got tired of walking, he would just sit and wait for any transportation offered by the Truffits. Begging for handouts could not be described as a way of life for Salty. More aptly it should be explained as his sole function of existence. The West Highland Terrier would sit at the right-hand side of his master at the dinner table and beg for morsels. The only way that Mr. Truffit could break his dog's concentrated stare was to accommodate him with a tidbit off his dinner plate. This offering would be repeated many times when they sat down for a meal. Besides handouts, Salty was fed canned food morning and night and had a dog pan full of dry food of which he could partake at his leisure. He did have to waddle into the service porch for the water and food—his only exercise. His poor little legs trying to hold up his enormous belly could be likened to a card table trying to hold up an automobile.

The Truffits were concerned about Salty's problem. Most of the time he could not make it outside by himself to take care of his nature calls. He had to be carried. They did not always anticipate his needs on time and he was having accidents in the house. "Our house is beginning to smell like an outside privy," was Mrs. Truffit's remark. "He is better than a garbage disposal. He will eat anything we call food and convert it into fat and waste. His waste products are a concern."

Obviously changes needed to be made. I was certain that I could not discuss Salty's problem graciously. Both members of the Truffit family were far from being slender. My approach to discuss this issue was a delicate matter. Tact was necessary.

"You are killing your Westie with love!" I continued by saying, "You are feeding him to death." I had the feeling in the first five to ten seconds that they would grab their dog from the exam table and stalk out of the hospital. Whatever I said about Salty could also be applied to their stature. They were obviously embarrassed by my remark and I knew that they did not enjoy the condition that they were in. I felt the major problem was a lack of self-control. I said a silent prayer and asked the Lord to guide me through the next few minutes of conversation. I proceeded.

"If you don't want Salty's fat engine to run all of the time, let's cut down on some of the fuel that runs it." I jiggled a handful of adipose tissue on the Westie's belly to demonstrate what I was referring to. My conversation continued. "Why don't you put a heaping tablespoon of canned diet food in four different locations in the house far enough away so that he has to get some exercise in order to satisfy his insatiable appetite. Do this twice daily so he will consume a total of one-half can at each feeding. Place the water pan next to the back door for a total of five locations. Since you have a yard, leave Salty outside most of the time—particularly when it is your mealtime. If Saltie does not walk, he does not eat." I was counting on the Westie to have an insatiable hunger and finally get off his rump and search for food once he realized where his meals were located. Hopefully, he would establish an eating route. Maybe this plan would work. "No tidbits, leftovers, or any hand-outs whatsoever should be offered to him no matter how much he begs. Allow him only an hour in the house at a time and fix him a bed outside by the back door."

Mr. and Mrs. Truffit were shifting their weight from one foot to the other and feeling guilty. I had unintentionally pointed my finger at them as well. I explained that Salty was controlling them—not the reverse. At that moment, I felt uncomfortable for I had overdone it a bit and come on too strong. I didn't look them in the eye for I felt a bit guilty approaching the problem as I had.

My next suggestion was to chart Salty's progress at home. Write down each bit of food offered to him. Record his weight daily if possible. I wanted to see Salty every other week to check his progress. I dispensed a daily vitamin for the Truffits to give Salty. Jo had overheard some of my discussion and just shook her head as the Truffits exited my hospital. The seventeenth of the month came and went. The Truffits had missed their appointment. I had Jo call to reschedule. No one was at home. Jo reminded me that I probably had been too dogmatic in my remarks about obesity and that the Truffits were unlikely to ever come here again. I explained to Jo that that was very possible. Each of us can shop around until we like what we hear. If we get twenty "no's" to one "yes" and we are searching for a "yes," it is human nature to bond to the person who agrees with one's thinking. My intention was basically sound but my approach left something to be desired. Jo phoned for the next few days and received no response. We laid the matter to rest.

The following Wednesday when I returned from my Rotary Club luncheon, the Truffits were waiting in the reception room with Salty. I hadn't seen them for a month. They said that Salty had not lost very much weight but that he was now walking from one food dish to the other. "We keep him outside most of the time and once he realized that we were not going to let him in the house, he quit his yapping at the back door. All of our carpets have been cleaned and our house smells nice enough again to invite guests over."

The Truffits were all smiles and for obvious reasons—they had lost a noticeable amount of weight themselves. I complimented them on their new look and Salty's progress. They shared with me that they had read the book *How to Win At Losing* and decided to change their eating style. To make it easier for them to accomplish this they left the house for about a month mainly to escape from their refrigerator. They had reevaluated their own eating habits and had adhered to a new plan. Their change helped their Westie as well. He was not inside when they ate and the old adage of "out of sight, out of mind" worked. Mrs. Truffit said, "We started taking short walks with Salty around the block. We now take a walk daily rather than nine trips to the refrigerator. When we feel like a snack we take a walk to remove the temptation. We walk slowly to accommodate Salty's pace."

Jo smiled at me as the three left the hospital and said, "I am glad that they came back."

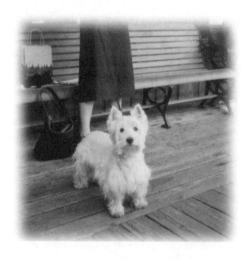

# —10—

# DOC ON THE SPOT

I said good-by to my sons, gave Marna a kiss, and headed for my car. As I backed out of the driveway, I noticed Allen and George walking down the street toward school. The morning was not spectacular in any great sense but there was a freshness in the air pushed inland by a gentle sea breeze. The salt air refreshed me, enabled me to take my mind off of my anticipated hospital routine, and compelled me to enjoy the beginning of the Lord's day.

My eyes were transfixed on the road ahead and my thoughts were dulled by the morning's routine trip to the office. I became alert because of some erratic drivers ahead. A car had stopped in the middle of the road and another car was stopped near it at a crazy angle. I suspected that the two drivers had met unexpectedly and were stopped to investigate the damages to their vehicles. I quickly found that I was wrong.

In the middle of the street was a dog. Several persons were standing nearby and a man said that he would drag the dog off to the side of the street so that other cars would not run over it. At that time, I stepped up and identified myself as a veterinarian. Immediately I was in charge as the spectators stepped back and allowed me to take over. I checked the brown and white comatose dog in front of me—he was still alive. I asked for a towel or blanket and a board or something stiff to use as a stretcher. An old towel appeared first and then a piece of heavy cardboard. I was just sliding the injured Springer Spaniel up on the makeshift stretcher when the local police arrived.

Someone had called in about an accident and the officer had responded. The officer used his patrol car with lights flashing to block that portion of the street and then directed those persons standing around to disperse. I asked an attentive lady if she knew the owner. She said, "I've seen the dog before, but do not know who it belongs to." The officer helped me carry the injured dog to my car and both of us then went our separate ways.

Jo saw me pull into the parking lot and stop near the front door. I beckoned to her to come out and help me. We proceeded to carry our patient into the treatment room and place him on the table. There was no collar or anything to identify either the dog or his owner. He was very pale. I attached the intravenous system and commenced a drip of plasma expander on one leg and saline and dextrose on the other leg. Solu-delta-cortef was added to counteract shock. I wondered what else would be feasible to do without the owner's permission. I decided to take an X ray while the Springer was still comatose and could be positioned properly. I had just stepped out of the darkroom with the wet film when Jo came in and said that the owner of the pet was out front and wanted to see her dog. "She is rather insistent and wants to see Spock now!"

I asked Jo to bring the owner back to the treatment room. Mrs. Arness was in tears. She had dropped her children off at school and then stopped at the grocery store before heading home. By word of mouth through her neighborhood watch she had been identified as the owner. When she pulled into her driveway, she noted a lady knocking on her front door. In my haste I had neglected to leave a business card or anything to enable her to locate me, but someone must have recognized me for the first place she came was to my hospital.

We looked at the radiograph together and I explained my interpretation. Spock had a diaphragmatic hernia. Considerable blood had pooled in the abdominal cavity and this indicated that he had received a major blow to his body. Other injuries might have occurred also. I explained what I had already done. She thanked me and requested that I do all I can to save Spock.

Jo and the owner went to the front desk and Jo recorded the owner's name, address, and other pertinent data about the owner and the pet. Spock was a four-year-old male Springer Spaniel, brown and white in color. I asked Jo to shift the morning appointments for a couple of hours. Triage was necessary. Whole blood was required, so I stopped the blood expander for the moment and connected a pint of whole blood to the intravenous drip system. Spock's belly was clipped and scrubbed and our patient was taken into surgery. Gas anesthetic could be added at our discretion when and if needed.

The telephone was ringing constantly that morning and I felt I would need uninterrupted help in surgery, so I had Jo call Marna to come down. Marna arrived all dressed up, heels and all. I remembered she had a baby shower to attend but faithfully she had responded to my request for assistance. Marna now took over the reception desk and Jo came back to assist me in surgery.

I made a ventral midline incision at the linea alba of the abdominal wall and immediately blood flowed out through the incision. I extended the incision and packed off the area with sponges in order to obtain a better view of the problem. There was a large rent in the spleen. The spleen needed to be repaired or removed before I could even consider correcting the hernia. I made the decision to proceed with a splenectomy. I double clamped all of the vessels connected to the spleen and then cut between the forceps. This freed the spleen from the body and I lifted it from the confines of Spock's abdomen. The free blood in the abdominal cavity was soaked up with gauze sponges and then I tied off the remaining vessels that were still clamped by the forceps. As each vessel was ligated, I removed the forceps. Soon I had an area where I could see the diaphragm and tend to that problem.

The tear in the diaphragm was sutured closed and negative pressure was again reestablished in the thoracic cavity. The abdomen was carefully checked for any further damage. No other problems existed and the ventral midline incision was closed. Spock was then bandaged securely around his middle. We carried him into critical care with both the intravenous and the oxygen supplies connected. The transfusion was almost complete so I instructed Jo to reconnect the plasma expander when the entire unit of blood had been administered.

I glanced at my watch and it was ten minutes after eleven. I had been in surgery almost two hours. It was time to have Jo return to the front desk and for Marna to make an appearance at her party.

The reception room was full of clients and their pets. Jo had both exam rooms occupied by the time I had shed my surgical gown and put on a smock. I then went to work. The clients were very understanding about the delay and that relieved me of a lot of stress. Fifteen minutes later Marna walked into the hospital with sandwiches and drinks. She knew both Jo and I would be busy through the noon hour and had been kind enough to bring us lunch.

# –11–

## LOOSE CAT

**S**unday morning had arrived and I was up early. Four hospitals plus my own were on my schedule for treatments that Memorial Day weekend. I planned to check the cases at my Redondo Beach hospital first before visiting two in Torrance, one in Hawthorne, and the last in San Pedro. This route was established in the hopes of meeting Marna and the boys at church.

I had only four animals at my hospital. Two were post-surgery cases and they were doing fine. Another needed an antibiotic injection to help reduce its fever and the last was being kenneled over the long holiday weekend. All of my employees had plans for the three-day weekend and had asked to be relieved of their responsibilities. Therefore, I needed to feed the pets, clean their cages, and give them fresh water. When this was completed, I headed east to one of the Torrance hospitals.

The kennel staff had not yet arrived and I needed assistance on several cases. I pulled the patient records and lined them up on the counter in the order I planned to treat them. Two of the patients were abscesses and the felines needed to be restrained in order to lavage their wounds and infuse ointment. Another cat had not been eating and gruel needed to be pumped into its stomach using a stomach tube. I was having considerable difficulty trying to treat the patients for it took skill to avoid their front claws when they refused to cooperate. Finally the kennel staff arrived and I solicited one of them to assist. The three cats were treated according to their needs. Next a dog required my attention and the kennel man brought it in. It was large and unmanageable so the second attendant was also required. The dog had been in a fight and acted like it still wanted to get even. We finally had to muzzle it to insure our safety. His neck had been sutured and all looked well there. His flank had also been tended to and sported a bandage to keep him from chewing at the lesion. Somehow he had been able to reach his back leg and nose or chew the bandage so the lesion was uncovered enabling him to have a clear shot at the sutures. Six of the seven had been chewed out and they needed to be replaced. I scrubbed the leg, blocked the lesion with xylocaine, and replaced the sutures. The leg was rebandaged, but I knew that the dog would not leave it alone so I placed a plastic collar on him to shield the bandaged leg from his attention.

I checked the rest of the cases in the hospital for temperature, pulse, and respiration as well as giving them a cursory examination. When the last patient had been seen, I filed the patient cards in the hospital rack and headed for my second Torrance location, which was only about a mile away.

The staff had already arrived and in a few minutes I was busy treating the cases. One case, a large calico cat, did not wish to cooperate. She was a terror and very difficult to get out of her cage. By the time two or three of us struggled to get her on the treatment table, she was hyper. I instructed one of the staff to put on a pair of heavy leather gloves that her teeth could not penetrate. Carefully we put her into a restraining sleeve that is somewhat like a long tube where her head could stick out. There were zippers all over the sleeve so all we had to do was unzip the appropriate place and treat that exposed area. This worked very well. The zipper over her right front leg was opened and the abscess treated. Antibiotics were given and she was returned to her cage.

My assistant took the calico cat to her cage in the canvas sleeve and unzipped it to let her out. When she was free of her restrainer, she made a beeline for open space. She went under his arm and escaped before he could get the cage door closed. From the treatment room, I heard "loose cat." Others heard it in the hospital and we all reacted in the same manner. All of the doors in the hospital were immediately closed. Now our precious little calico ball of fire was confined and fortunately the area of her restriction was her own ward.

Calico crouched in the corner of the ward and her head was so low to the floor that we could not lasso her with a leash. To add to the problem, she would bat the leash away with either foot if we were about to succeed. None of us wanted to be either scratched or bitten so we had to be very cautious. I put on the leather gloves and tried to capture her but when I got down that low, I could not maneuver with any agility. Each time I would reach for her she would jump toward my face. We all agreed that another method had to be employed to recage the terrified cat.

We retired to another part of the hospital to concoct a plan and let the cat calm down some. When we returned to implement it, the calico cat was not there. She had jumped back into her own cage. We shut the door amid a sigh of relief. Apparently she felt more secure in the confines of her cage than out in the open spaces of the floor where large humans had been trying to "rope" her.

I still had another hospital to visit. I thanked the staff for their assistance and headed north to Hawthorne. They had five borders for me to check plus several cases to treat. The staff brought in the nontreatment cases first and appropriate entries were made on their patient cards.

I changed the intravenous drip on a car accident case and rechecked the positioning of the splint on the rear leg. There was a note on the cage for me to please recheck this case both afternoon and evening. A cat needed medication applied to its right eye as well as an antibiotic injection. Another case had been put into the metabolic cage in order to collect urine. Urine had been collected so I did a cursory laboratory test with urostix and gave the remainder to a staff member to be set aside for a more extensive analysis at a local laboratory. I asked my assistant to call and see if the sample could be picked up on Sunday.

Church service was already in progress and I knew that I wouldn't be able to meet Marna and the boys there. We had previously agreed on a location for brunch after the treatments at my hospital. If I was too late for church, I had planned to meet my family there after I had completed all the treatment cases that morning.

I had brunch with Marna and the boys and returned home to take a nap. I had been up a good bit of the night and had started early that morning. I even decided to forgo my supper and continue my nap. I would eat later. Marna had advised the boys to be extra quiet as Daddy was sleeping. Marna fed the boys in the kitchen as that was the farthest place from my slumber area. I didn't hear the phone ring but opened my eyes when George gently shook my shoulder and announced that the Manhattan Beach operator was on the line.

I stumbled into the kitchen and picked the phone off the counter. A young man named Crawford had just run over his dog's foot with a power lawn mower. His pet's foot was bleeding badly and his neighbor would chauffeur him to the hospital since his parents were not at home. I recommended that he wrap the injured foot in a towel or some other clean cloth and head for the hospital. Marna had made a meatloaf for supper and after hearing my telephone conversation, quickly made a sandwich and handed it to me as I headed out the door.

John Crawford and his neighbor arrived with Pooch. We went into the treatment room and I unwrapped the bleeding foot. John turned pale and became nauseous. His neighbor took over the responsibility of lending me a hand. I covered the rear right foot again and filled a syringe with surital and then administered it intravenously to quiet Pooch down and take away the pain. I went outside and brought in the anesthetic machine and passed John who had taken refuge in a chair in the reception room. His face was buried in his hands and he was crying.

Pooch was now breathing the anesthetic and under my complete control. I opened the cloth around his foot again and evaluated the badly mangled foot. Pieces of bone were exposed so I carried Pooch into the X-ray room and took several views. When the radiographs had been developed, I went out front to discuss the evidence with the boy and his neighbor. John did not want to look at the film and neither did the neighbor who told me to go ahead and do whatever was necessary to save the foot. I realized how stressed both of them were by this time so I returned to the back of the hospital to help the dog.

I transferred Pooch to surgery and then placed the film on the view screen. Two toes had been severed and the other two had been stripped of flesh in many places. I had a lot of work to do so I advised the neighbor to take John home and wait for my phone call after surgery was completed. They left and I locked the front door behind them.

I scrubbed up and put on a surgical gown and gloves. The two mangled toes were amputated. On the two damaged digits I was able to reconstruct the tissue and only hoped that there was enough blood supply to enable them to be saved. An hour and a half later I took off my gloves and removed the drapes that had protected the surgical site. The foot looked pretty good and I felt that it had a good chance to recover.

I called John at his home. His neighbor answered. He had stayed with John until I called. John did not want to come to the phone and I understood for the twelve-year-old boy had just gone through a very traumatic experience.

The neighbor who had just identified himself as Kevin said that he would relay John's questions to me.

"John wants to know if Pooch lost his foot?"

"No, I think we can save it—but time will tell."

"Can he walk on it?"

"I think he could but I would prefer he didn't"

"What's going to happen now and when can he go home?"

"I am going to wrap the leg and pad it with ample cotton in order to cushion it so the toes can be protected. About going home, I plan to leave that to your regular veterinarian who will make that decision in the morning. Pooch is still recovering from his anesthetic so he will definitely stay overnight."

"John told me that Pooch chases the mower and barks at it. John was trying to mow the lawn in a hurry before it got dark. When he turned the mower around to go back, he surprised Pooch who couldn't get completely out of the way."

"I'll bet Pooch keeps clear of the mower from now on," I said.

"Hopefully he won't have to do it on only three legs," was the response.

It was Monday morning of the Memorial Day weekend and it was necessary for me to visit the same hospitals that I had done on Sunday and check the pets that needed care. At the Torrance hospital, I watched the attendant, wearing leather gloves, carefully open Calico's cage and reach in for her. Calico hissed but allowed the gloves to encompass her and she was lifted out of her cage and placed on the table in the exam room. The leather gloves were surrounding her neck like a wide stiff collar, immobilizing her. I was able to treat her foot and exercised caution. She was returned to her cage and as soon as she was released, she attempted to attack her handler but it was too late for the cage door had been securely closed. The other staff member was supposed to have placed food and water in Calico's cage while the cage was vacant but had neglected to do so. I now watched as the cage was again carefully opened and a water pan was slid into her cage followed by her morning food dish. Calico had backed up into the corner and snarled as all of this activity took place. I completed the last of my treatment cases and headed for San Pedro.

All of the staff had come and gone. A couple of notes were on the counter. One note said that I should not try to take the German Shepherd from his cage as he is rather mean and hard to rekennel. I noted on his card that his ears had already been treated by the staff. I appreciated their thoughtfulness. The second note asked me to call a client that had an emergency and needed to see me when I arrived. I called the Lennox house and asked them to bring Pico right down. I was able to treat the balance of the cases before they arrived.

Mrs. Lennox arrived just as I was caging my last treatment case. She was a client of the hospital so I located her card from the file. I noted that she owned four cats and two dogs. She had brought in Pico, a gray and white, short-hair, altered male cat.

Pico was crouched in the back of his cage so I gently lifted him out and placed him on a towel. He objected slightly when I moved his right rear leg. Mrs. Lennox said, "He had been outside and had come to the back door and cried to come in. He then limped across the floor and got on his favorite pillow in the kitchen and seemed content to just stay there. He is not interested in food, in fact he has eaten nothing since he entered the house and that is not like him. He objects when anyone tries to pick him up. I believe there is something seriously wrong with his right rear leg."

I checked him carefully and he cried when I moved his rear end to insert the thermometer. I checked his feet and his front claws were flayed. This indicated to me that he probably had been hit by a car. Cats flying out of control through the air extend their claws in an attempt to grab something to stop their flight and when they hit the road or some concrete, they tatter their front claws.

Permission was granted to take several X rays. I brought the wet films out to the view screen and we perused them together. Nothing significant was noted in the abdominal area but the pelvic view showed considerable trauma. There was a separation in the pelvic symphysis and the right femur was fractured. I had already given the cat a mild sedative in order to position Pico properly for the radiographs, so I was able to structure and fit a protective splint to insure that the sharp ends of the fractured femur would not cause further damage. An injection was given for shock. I explained that surgery would probably be done on Tuesday morning because we wanted to evaluate the possibility of any internal injuries that might be present but not evident at this time.

Mrs. Lennox wanted to carry Pico to his cage in the hospital ward. I proceeded to prepare the cage and then invited Mrs. Lennox to bring Pico back and place him on several soft towels. She petted Pico and headed for home.

The treatment cases were taken care of at the other hospitals and I headed for the restaurant where Marna and the boys were waiting. Before I left my last clinic, I called the four answering services and gave them the telephone number where I could be located. It was always a pleasure to eat out with my family on holidays. I walked into the restaurant and Allen waved to me. They had already ordered brunch and were in the midst of eating it but were eating slowly in hopes that I would arrive while they were still there. When I placed my order, I told the waitress that I might have an emergency call so she would know where to find me.

I had not finished eating when the hostess came over and told me that I had a telephone call. I returned to the table and told them I needed to go back to San Pedro. George asked to go with me and Marna nodded. Albert wanted to go too but I felt that one son was enough. George and I quickly left and the Mustang was pointed south once again.

Mr. Avakian and his son were waiting for me when George and I arrived. Their German Shepherd is an aggressive dog and had gotten into another fight. On King's side and shoulder were several bite wounds. The entire area was covered with saliva, debris, and oozing blood. Considerable debris had collected there during his skirmish with the other dog. The area needed to be cleaned up so I could evaluate what needed to be done. I gave Mr. Avakian two choices. I could spot bathe King or I could put him into the tub and give him a complete bath before I did surgery. I suggested the latter. He agreed.

While I was bathing King, Mr. Avakian located a magazine in the reception room. George and the Avakian boy, Chuck, hit it off. George asked if he could show Chuck through the hospital and I said, "Yes, but be very quiet when you are in the wards because I don't want any of the patients to be disturbed and start barking." When King's bath was completed and he was toweled down, I called Mr. Avakian in and showed him two lacerations that would require suturing. George returned and held King's vein off and I injected sufficient surital to relax him completely.

I proceeded swiftly with the surgery as the anesthetic would only last ten minutes or so. I clipped the area and George vacuumed up the loose hair. I painted the surgical site with red zephrine, an antiseptic, and then draped it. The two lesions were debrided and then sutured. King was trying to raise his head when I secured the final stitch. I invited Mr. Avakian and Chuck in to inspect the surgery before I put King in a large recovery cage George had prepared for him. I was overruled by the owner who said that King may be unmanageable when he fully recovered.

With safety in mind for anyone who might have to handle King, I bent to Mr. Avakian's recommendation and helped him carry King out to his car and place him carefully on the back seat. His son stayed in the car to keep King company and we returned to the hospital to take are of the finances.

George was on the phone. The Manhattan Beach hospital was on the line. I asked George to tell them that I would call right back. Mr. Avakian left and I returned the call. The Manhattan Beach hospital was about fifteen miles away so I set a time to meet the client there so that neither one of us would have long to wait. George asked me what was the nature of the emergency and I told him that we were going to see a Mr. Onstad who had a poodle with a swollen face. We arrived at the same time as the client. George held the door open for him and the owner was instructed to go immediately into the exam room by my son. I picked up a blank client/patient card and filled it out as I asked for the pertinent information.

I took Daisy's temperature and it was higher than normal. On the side of her face was a large delineated swelling. I informed him that Daisy had an infected upper tooth. When Mr. Onstad questioned my diagnosis, I raised Daisy's cheek and applied gentle pressure to the swelling on her face. We all observed purulent matter being exuded between the gum and the tooth in question.

Mr. Onstad left the required deposit and departed. George carried Daisy into the treatment room while I went out to the Mustang to recover the anesthetic machine. George held Daisy and soon we were ready for dental surgery. The tooth was first extracted. Then the abscess pocket on her cheek was lanced before establishing a seton drain to facilitate future treatment and drainage of the infected area. George prepared a cage while I gave antibiotics and infused forte ointment into the abscessed area.

It was almost four in the afternoon when we pulled into the driveway at home. George exhibited unlimited energy and joined his brothers in the backyard for a game of catch. My goal was first to enjoy a glass of iced tea and then take a nap. However, two more emergencies occurred and I checked several hospital cases before calling it a night. It had been a long three-day holiday weekend for me.

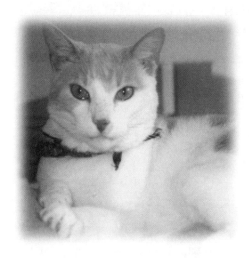

# 12-

# A GOOD CLIENT

**I** had shortchanged my last client. I did not realize what I had done until Jo brought it to my attention. My clients deserve the very best from me and Miss Corey just didn't receive it. The preceding client had really disturbed me. She had questioned everything I had done. My selection of medication, the dosage, where I planned to administer it, and so on. When I had finished taking care of her pet, I just wasn't in a good mood. She had taxed my patience to the utmost.

Unfortunately I had allowed my feelings to carry over to the next client which was Miss Corey. The flavor of a bunch of sour grapes still lingered in my mouth when Miss Corey and Bimini entered the exam room. I couldn't recall even smiling once and I made no effort to engage her in any small talk. Looking back, I wish I could reenact the office visit and be more cordial.

Bimini had a topknot held in place by a blue ribbon. He was a lively Yorkie pup and stood on the table wagging his tail and just begging for attention. Bimini gave a slight squeal as I inserted the thermometer. He was very attentive as I continued his initial examination. Miss Corey had an armful of questions that I should have taken time to respond to but instead I gave her a cold shoulder and handed her a booklet that contained most of the answers she had sought. My tableside manners had deteriorated markedly.

55

When Miss Corey had called for an appointment, Jo had instructed her to bring in a stool sample. She handed it to me and I, in turn, handed it to Jo who would do the laboratory work. Bimini was vaccinated with a combined vaccine that contained distemper, parvovirus, leptospirosis [a disease that affects the kidneys], and hepatitis. I handed her some sample vitamins and exited the exam room. Jo made an appointment for two weeks hence for the second vaccine and asked Miss Corey to call in a couple of hours for the results of the fecal examination.

She did make an appointment for the second vaccine and the fecal determination turned out to be negative for parasites. However, in ten days she called back and cancelled that appointment. Jo phoned several times and was able to only leave reminder messages on her answering device. Jo admonished me for losing a good client. I was sensitive to Jo's comment and this was haunting my conscience.

Two days after her appointment had been originally scheduled, Miss Corey was able to return Jo's phone call. She apologized for having to cancel the appointment. She was employed by Delta Airlines and had been out of town. She wanted to come down right away because she was leaving the next day on an early morning flight. Miss Corey arrived within the hour and Jo squeezed her in to my schedule just before a surgery.

Miss Corey arrived in a flight attendant's uniform. She apologized for her missed appointment and any trouble it may have caused us. She then thanked me for waiting. Bimini was excited to see me and needed to be held in such a manner so that his nose could be kept out of my way.

She wanted to explain why she missed her appointment as she felt very bad about any inconvenience she may have caused me. "I was called in unexpectedly to fill in for a sick flight attendant and just forgot to phone you and reschedule." I felt much better after her remark and was happy to know that she had overlooked my earlier rudeness.

Miss Corey had read the information booklet that had been given her and had numerous questions. I spent extra time responding to her questions. I felt fortunate that I had some time to correct my ungracious first contact with such a delightful person.

About ten days later, I had an emergency call from my hospital. It was almost two in the morning. The answering service for my hospital said that a Miss Wingate needed to talk to me. The operator patched me through. I introduced myself and asked what kind of problem her pet had.

Miss Wingate said that Sheila Corey had recommended me. "Sheila and I came in on a late flight and when I got home my cat seemed sick. I called Sheila and she gave me your name and phone number." After hearing her describe the symptoms, I agreed to meet her at my hospital in Redondo Beach. As I headed for my hospital, I had the opportunity to reflect and realize what a good client Miss Corey has been. I had not treated her very well initially but she had overlooked my faults and even recommended me to a friend.

Miss Wingate placed Mac upon the examination table. Mac was a tiger-striped short-hair male, who was straining to urinate. I checked his abdomen and the bladder was enlarged and tense. When I applied pressure no urine was expelled. I explained the need to give a short acting anesthetic and open the urethra to allow the urine to flow. I was given permission to proceed and she left. I locked the front door behind her and returned to the treatment room.

Mac was given surital intravenously and soon he was reclining on the treatment table. Using a special adapter, I attached it to a large syringe full of sterile saline and was able to successfully back flush the urethra blockage into the bladder. Now the urine could be expelled through the adapter by applying pressure to Mac's abdomen. When the bladder was void of urine, I inserted a catheter and anchored it in place with a suture to temporarily alleviate a repeat problem.

I cleaned up and headed for home. I had a contented client in Miss Corey or she would not have referred a client to me. I realized that no matter how much money is spent on advertising, it is impossible to buy or keep good clients. The best referral I can get is the recommendation from a satisfied client. A good table-side manner will determine whether my practice is a success or a failure and I was now well aware of that fact.

# —13—

## A NEW DOG

**I** had my elbow on the counter and was chatting with Jo, waiting for my last clients of the day to arrive. The Truffits had been gone all summer as they had driven across the United States in their motor home and had taken Salty with them. We wondered if all three of them had continued to lose weight or if the good start had gone asunder. They pulled into the parking lot and got out of their car. Jo said, "Look at them. They look like new people!" Jo suggested we have some fun with them so when they entered the hospital, Jo said, "May I have your name, please." Both the Truffits laughed and Mrs. Truffit remarked, "We haven't changed that much, have we?" Both Jo and I complimented them on their continued weight loss. Salty too had lost more weight, and I asked Jo to put him on the scales in the treatment room.

Mr. Truffit handed Jo the leash and Salty scampered eagerly into the rear of the hospital with Jo. That was the most action I had seen from Salty since I first met him. Jo returned and said that he weighed thirty-four pounds. That was a far cry from the fifty-seven pounds we had recorded earlier. Salty's diet had been in force long enough to exhibit an influence on the quality of his coat. Mrs. Truffit said, "Even the odor from his skin in gone!" They were right. Salty smelled better— the room smelled better. We were informed that Salty was kept outside most of the time and was using a specific area of the lawn exclusively for his potty area.

I felt that it was a blessing to have good clients who were willing to follow my suggestions. They shared with us that their neighbors are more friendly and often stop them when they are walking and visit with them. Mrs. Truffit said, "We go out more often and enjoy life more."

I was just closing the front door and heading home for the day when the phone rang. I lingered to see if it was for me. Jo handed me the phone and informed me that San Pedro was on the line. The operator patched me in to the Holbrooks.

The Holbrooks had been gone for a few days and when they got home and went to unpack and hang up some of their clothes, Kinko staggered out of the closet. They realized that their cat, Kinko, must have been confined there since they left. Kinko was very weak and needed to be hospitalized. I explained that I was not their regular doctor and would have to drive from Redondo Beach. "We'll be waiting for you," was their reply and then they hung up. I asked Jo to call Marna and tell her to go ahead to the dinner party and I would meet her there later.

The Holbrooks were waiting for me when I arrived at the hospital. I pulled their card from the files and we went into the exam room. Kinko's temperature, pulse, and respiration were normal but she was so weak that she was almost walking sideways. I rolled in the intravenous stand and started a slow drip of 5 percent saline and dextrose as well as sixty milliliters of the same solution under the skin at the nape of her neck. The amount that was administered subcutaneously would be a back-up nutritional supply as it would be absorbed into her system much more slowly than the intravenous solution.

"A teenager in the neighborhood was supposed to feed and water Kinko while we went to Chicago. We had talked to her initially about possibly putting Kinko into a kennel, so when she could not find Kinko she supposed that is what we had done. I guess that we did not communicate with her regarding our final decision."

I decided that Kinko would receive excellent care at home so I explained that small feedings of canned cat food every two or three hours would be best. When she was satisfied, they could then feed her larger quantities and leave food out for her the way they usually did. They thanked me for driving across town and we left together.

I finally arrived at the dinner party. The dinner was to be on the veranda where we had a spectacular view of San Pedro Harbor. Before I could locate Marna, three elderly lady friends who moved in our same social circle cornered me and wanted to know what I had been doing. They had heard from Marna that I was out on an emergency and they were inquisitive. I briefly explained the reason for my delay but found it impossible to disengage myself from the conversation. I would have given Marna our prearranged rescue signal, but she was nowhere in sight. Marna probably didn't even know I had arrived otherwise she would have been at my side.

I was relieved when the hostess came by and suggested we find our designated tables as dinner was about to be served. I knew that Marna would soon appear so I lingered for a moment at the table to seat her. Marna arrived at the same time the caterer began pouring the champagne. She reminded me that it was a fiftieth anniversary party and that she had taken care of finding an appropriate card.

I was interrupted twice that evening by phone falls. Both could be handled without leaving the party. It was nice to attend a social function with Marna and be there the entire time—almost. I had just taken my first bite of wedding cake when a neighbor who was at the party came over and whispered in my ear that one of his children had just called and said that their dog, Skipper, had just collapsed and appeared dead. "Could you come next door and take a look?" I asked Marna to get the anesthetic machine from my Mustang and I left immediately for the neighbor's house.

Skipper was on the living room floor just where he had fallen. I checked his chest and could feel a heartbeat. His tongue was a sickly gray. He did not respond to any reflexes. Just then Marna arrived pushing in the oxygen setup. She had been wise enough to bring in a selection of tracheal tubes so I selected the proper one and intubated Skipper. The color of Skipper's mucous membranes improved and his pulse became stronger. I stood up and turned to say something to the owner. When I turned to look at the inflatable oxygen bag on the machine, the bag was no longer inflating. I checked the pulse again and there was none. Skipper had just experienced a terminal heart attack.

Thank goodness I had my machine in the car's trunk. I had used it on an emergency of this nature for the first time, but it was to no avail. My patient did not survive. I rolled the anesthetic machine out to the car and disassembled it again so it could fit in the trunk. Marna left for home and I followed. Our three sons were fast asleep. I paid the sitter and then looked at Marna. We were both wide awake so we ended the evening with a cup of fresh brewed coffee while we recapped our evening's experience.

# —14—

# DECISION TIME

I had decided to replace a window pane rather than take a nap. An errant throw of a baseball by one of the boys had caused the problem. The boys were more than willing to help. Allen went to the garage for the ladder, George found a bucket for the shards of glass and Albert volunteered to help pick up the pieces of glass that adorned the ground under the window. The rest of the broken glass was removed from the window and the edges of the window frame were cleared of the old putty and glazing points. I had just positioned the new pane of glass and affixed it to the window frame when the telephone rang. The Gardena operator had Mrs. Ureda on the line and she wanted me to meet her at the Gardena hospital because her Pekinese had a very sore foot. We agreed to meet in an hour. I returned to my window job and put on the glazing putty and then asked the boys to put the ladder away and clean up the rest of the mess for me. They assured me that the task would be completed before I returned home.

I pulled the Ureda card and went into the exam room. I noted a little red star in the corner of the card and heeded the warning. Nipper was obviously a little cantankerous. I took a long look at his moniker and realized he had been well named.

Nipper had a coat full of foxtails and when I noticed the wet and swollen area of his front paw where he had been licking, it was easy to make my diagnosis—an interdigital foxtail abscess. I asked Mrs. Ureda to carry Nipper into the treatment room and restrain him while he was sedated with surital. Soon he was lying peaceably on the table. Mrs. Ureda wanted to know if she could comb out Nipper's coat while he was sedated because it was impossible to do when he was awake. I said that it would be alright for her to do that as soon as I had completed the foot surgery.

I lanced the abscess by extending the point of penetration of the foxtail. After a little bit of probing, I soon held the foxtail in the grip of my alligator forceps. I took it out to the front room and showed it to the owner. Then I invited her to follow me back to do the grooming that she had requested.

After several minutes, Mrs. Ureda had made very little progress with the comb and brush that I had provided. I knew that the job she had commenced had no chance of being completed before Nipper recovered from the sedative. I suggested that it may be more practical to close clip Nipper all over leaving only the head and tail long. "This clipping style should last all summer and his coat will grow out again in the fall," was my suggestion. She readily agreed that my idea was sensible. I escorted her to the front door and locked her out after informing her that Nipper would stay the night and have his bath in the morning.

Nipper was waking up more each minute so I titered him with some more of the surital that was still in the syringe taped to his foot. He received a close clip. The head and tail were left unclipped and that left me the job of combing them out. Normally I would have left him for the morning staff to bathe as I had told Mrs. Ureda, but the little red star on his card made me think twice. It is always much easier to bathe and rinse a standing pet than one in a prone position but Nipper could be very difficult to handle in the morning. I put on a waterproof apron and gave him a thorough bath, rinsing, and toweling.

I filled in all of the data on the patient card and then made out a cage card with a prominent red star in the upper right corner. The premises were restored to order and I headed for home to inspect the boy's clean-up job.

Marna and I had just said goodnight to our boys and retired to the family room when the phone rang. The Manhattan Beach exchange had the Balsters on the line. They had a very sick cat. Mr. Balster was on the phone and said, "Mac Beth has been sick for the last two or three days and just seems to be getting worse by the minute. What do you think is the problem ?"

"Gosh, I don't know." I answered. "Is he eating?"

"No, not for two days."

"Is he interested in food at all?"

"No, he has just taken up residence on his favorite cushion and won't move."

"I think that I should see him."

"How much will it cost, doctor?"

I quoted the emergency and the examination fees. "Anything in addition to this will mean further charges which we can discuss when I see him and know what needs to be done."

"We live about ten minutes from you and can come right down."

"I am at home now and it will take me at least twenty minutes to get to the hospital if the traffic is favorable."

"Okay, we will be there in twenty minutes."

The Balsters were waiting when I arrived. I filled out the client/patient card before the examination. Mac Beth was a large tiger-striped male that normally would have weighed fifteen pounds. I was looking at a cat that was fur and bones and too weak to stand. I first inserted a thermometer and then reflected his eye lid. The sclera of his eye was a pronounced yellow. I checked his gums and they were yellow tinged. Mac Beth had jaundice. I then palpated his abdominal area and found a large mass in the anterior portion. I looked up at the Balsters who had been patiently waiting for my comment. They must have read my expression for Mr. Balster said, "It's pretty bad, isn't it?"

I said, "Yes, he has a large mass that is probably cancerous and very likely associated with his liver."

"Then there is not much hope."

"Not a lot, but where there's life there is always some hope. Is Mac Beth your only cat?"

"No, we have two other cats."

"It is not likely that he will pull through. Surgery and long term care must be considered."

"How much will it cost to put him under?"

I quoted the fee.

"Okay, doc, go ahead and do it."

They signed the necessary papers and I returned to the back of the hospital to do my task while they waited. When all was done, they wanted to say good-bye to Mac Beth so all of us went back for their farewells.

At the front desk, Mr. Balster handed me a few dollars and fished in his pocket for some change. Mrs. Balster rummaged through her purse for some additional funds. When all of the money was displayed on the counter, there was barely enough to cover the emergency fee let alone the examination or the euthanasia. Mr. Balster looked at me and said, "Doc, that's all we have till payday. I'll come in and pay more then." I reached over and picked up the five-dollar bill and told him that it would cover the hospital expense and we would call it even.

For a moment he just stood there and looked at me as tears welled up in his eyes. He said, "Much obliged." He picked up the remaining money from the counter. Mrs. Balster thanked me and they left. They pulled out of the driveway in their old car and waved at me as they passed the front door.

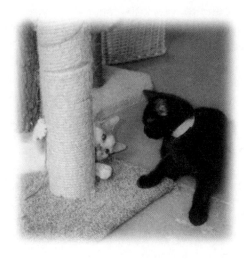

# —15—

# GOING VISITING

The boys were in front of the fireplace playing a board game. Marna and I were seated near the coffee table engaged in a game of cribbage. Greta was stretched out between the boys and the fire, constantly disturbing the board game whenever she stretched her legs. Faux Pas, our Siamese cat, was snuggled up on her favorite basket on the hearth. All was calm on the western front.

The ringing of the phone broke the silence. The Kronenburg's Labrador was badly cut and he needed to be sutured. I suggested that they wrap him up in a sheet or blanket to protect the car's upholstery from any bloodstains and head immediately for the Manhattan Beach hospital. I told them I would leave right away also.

The boys were involved in their game and each in turn declined to accompany me. I was saying good-bye when Marna said that she had not been asked to join me. I apologized and asked her along. She quickly grabbed her sweater and we left together.

Mr. Kronenburg lifted Barry, their black Labrador, out of their car and I hurriedly held open the front door while Marna turned on the lights. We went immediately into the treatment room where I inspected his injuries. There were two significant cuts on Barry. One across the underside of his abdomen and the other on the anterior portion of his rear leg just below the kneecap, or patella. Barry was bleeding from both of the lesions. Marna stayed with the clients in the treatment room and held pressure packs over both of the wounds while I brought in the anesthetic machine from the car. Barry was given a sedative, was intubated, and was now breathing gas.

Both of the Kronenburgs looked a little pale at the sight of the gapping wounds and the blood so I suggested they return to the reception room while I did the surgery. Marna was not comfortable helping me in surgery, but she did not complain when I asked her to assist. I could not locate the bleeders right away so Marna again applied pressure with some of the gauze sponges while I clipped the fur from around the lesions. I was finally able to locate the two prominent vessels and clamped them off. Most of the hemorrhaging ceased. I left the clamps in place while the surgical area was debrided and swabbed with an antiseptic. Surgical drapes were placed around the chest wound. The vessels that had previously been clamped were now tied off. Several smaller vessels that were discovered were cauterized electrically. All debris was removed and an antibiotic powder was puffed onto the raw tissue. Suturing followed and at least twenty stitches were required to complete the closure.

My next undertaking was to determine how much damage had occurred to Barry's leg. The cut was across his leg and the tendon that attached to his patella was partially severed. We prepared this surgical site as before. Little hemorrhaging was evident by this time. My main concern was the tendon. It needed to be strengthened with sutures before flexion severed it completely. Using a stainless steel suture and a figure-eight stitch, the edges of tendon were reunited again.

A splint was necessary for if Barry flexed his leg, the suture might pull through the sinews and all the surgery I had done would have been to no avail. A walking splint was fitted to the leg. A portion of old rubber inner tube was taped over the aluminum base of the splint to keep the splint from slipping as Barry walked.

I detached Barry from the anesthetic machine and gave him an injection of antibiotic to alleviate any possibility of infection. His color was good so I rationalized that a little bit of blood loss looks like an enormous amount when spread around over a large surface area. With this thought in mind I did not administer either a blood transfusion or a plasma expander.

Marna prepared a cage for Barry and then helped me carry him in and place him on several layers of terry cloth towels. We decided to clean up the surgery and treatment rooms next before we invited the Kronenburgs in because we felt that they were a bit squeamish regarding the sight of blood.

I put the surgery pack in the autoclave while Marna went out front to invite the clients to the recovery ward where Barry was located. I explained what damage had been done and how I had corrected Barry's injuries. I shared with them the reason for the necessity of a splint. We visited a bit and I fielded numerous questions regarding Barry's aftercare both here and after he is discharged. I gave Marna a glance and she received it promptly and invited the Kronenburgs to the reception desk where she recorded the anamnesis and other pertinent data on the medical card.

Marna returned and told me that the owners had been keeping Barry inside because the neighbor's dog was in heat. The attraction was too great for him and he had decided to jump out of a window and go visiting. They heard the window break and traced the bloody trail to the house next door. Even his injuries had not discouraged him on his adventure.

The autoclave bell rang and I vented the machine. When the pack was cool enough, I replaced it on the shelf. Marna was wondering if there was more to do. I asked her if she had made an appointment for a recheck. She had not but told me she asked the owners to make one when Barry was discharged.

As we stepped into the car, I mentioned to Marna that I had one more place to stop. That stop was at a local coffee shop where we enjoyed pie and coffee before heading home.

Early the next morning, I had reached for the phone on my nightstand and dropped it disconnecting the line. I put the phone back in its cradle and almost immediately it rang again. The operator from the Palos Verdes hospital was on the line and connected me to a concerned client. Mrs. Claymore was calling about Pepper, her miniature Schnauzer. "Pepper seems to have trouble urinating. He woke me up at 2 A.M., about an hour ago, and wanted to go outside. He came back in and before I got back to sleep, he wanted to go outside again. My husband followed him outside with a flashlight thinking that an opossum or raccoon may be in the yard. That wasn't the case at all. Pepper would go over to his favorite tree and raise his leg. He really did not urinate at all except for only a drop or two. He is very uncomfortable. Can I pick up some medication at your office this morning that will give him some relief?"

"It sound to me that Pepper needs some help right away. Can you meet me at the Palos Verdes hospital?"

Mrs. Claymore said, "I can be at your hospital at 3:30."

"I'll be waiting for you and Pepper."

I arrived ten minutes before the Claymores. Pepper was taken into the treatment room. I had already pulled his record card as he was a regular patient of that hospital. Pepper was still straining with no result. I attempted to pass a urinary catheter but it hit a blockage after only a short distance. An X ray was taken with the catheter in place and a urinary stone was quite visible in the urethra just past the tip of the catheter. I tried to back flush the stone into the bladder but the distended bladder was exerting too much pressure and the stone refused to dislodge. Surgery was now a necessity. The owners helped and soon an area had been clipped below his anus and dorsal to his scrotum. I brought in my anesthetic machine and connected Pepper. He was now under my control and breathing metafane gas.

I sent the Claymores home and told them I would call them after surgery. I set out the sterile equipment I needed, gloved up, and commenced surgery. A vertical incision was made ventral to the anus. The urethra was exposed just anterior to the cartilage penis and an incision was then made through the urethral wall. The urinary stone was milked out through the incision and followed almost immediately by a voluminous flow of urine. I could almost hear Pepper give a sigh of relief. I passed a catheter through the urethral incision into the bladder, expressed the bladder manually, and allowed the balance of the urine to be excreted. The stone was salvaged for a laboratory analysis and a sample of urine also set aside. It was not necessary to close either the urethral or skin incisions for they would heal on their own. Besides, if other stones were passed, they would find an easy exit for they could easily be expelled through the urethral incision before it healed.

I gave Pepper a couple of injections after the anesthetic was detached. A cage was prepared with ample towels to soak up any urine he discharged. The surgery pack was made up and put into the autoclave. The surgery room was restored to its normal cleanliness, and I then called the Claymores and reported to them regarding the surgery.

It was too late to go home. The sky was now light and the clock informed me it was almost half past five. I decided to have breakfast at a nearby restaurant and then go to my own hospital and shave and clean up before my clients started arriving.

Jo unlocked the front door when she arrived. She had noticed my car outside and knew that I had been busy during the night. Her first remark was: "Wow! You look like you have been up all night!"

# —16—

# A Drop-In Assistant

**M**arna stopped by the hospital to see if I had time to join her for lunch. I was busily engaged in correcting a prolapsed rectum in a cat when she stuck her head in the surgery door to see when I would be finished. Two clients were backed up waiting for me in the reception room so I informed Marna that it would be impossible this noon to spend any time with her.

I completed surgery and replaced my surgical gown with a clean smock. Now I was ready to see my two patients. I called on the inner phone line and asked Jo to put the waiting clients into the examination rooms. Marna answered. She had told Jo that she would pinch hit for her while she allowed Jo to go to lunch. I was very appreciative of Marna's willingness to assist at the hospital.

Vaccines were given to one patient and the other patient had the seton removed from an abscess. Soon they were on their way. Jo still had not returned so Marna did some filing while I organized the surgery and cleaned up the surgical instruments. When this task was completed, the surgical pack was placed in the autoclave for sterilization. Jo walked in the front door just as a car pulled into the parking lot and a man hurried into the hospital with an injured Chow dog.

He had hit the dog with his car and was kind enough to insure that the Chow had medical attention. He did not wish to take financial responsibility for the injured pet, but he pushed the required emergency fee at Marna and left without giving us any information other than the street where the accident occurred.

The Chow had sustained a head injury. There was a deep gash across the top of his head and a lot of hair was missing there. Most of the bleeding had stopped but whatever remained of a beautiful coat on his cranium was now a matted mass of fur and blood.

Jo looked at me. I looked at Marna. Marna put her purse back into my office and took over the front desk responsibilities again. Jo and I carried the Chow into treatment from the exam room. I checked my patient more thoroughly. The Chow was alert but exhibited signs of disorientation and seemed confused. He gave us the impression that he was looking right at us but couldn't see us. He was content to just lie there on his side and rest. Only his ears would move with any alertness for when either Jo or I spoke, it appeared that he was trying to listen to our conversation. When a bright light was shone into his eyes, his pupils did not restrict. Our patient had a concussion of an unknown magnitude.

An endotracheal tube was passed to insure the patient's air passageway. Jo trimmed and scrubbed his scalp and cleaned up the area for surgery. She painted the top of his head with red zephrine. A swelling was evident now just anterior to his right ear. Some decisions had to be made without the owner's permission.

Since the patient was semi-conscious, I decided to suture up the laceration across his skull. As I was suturing the wound, the Chow would flinch and his reaction became more pronounced with each suture. By the time I had finished, our black Chow was showing more response. He had been hit on the head and knocked out and I began to realize that the injury was only a mild concussion rather than a more severe one as I had first suspected.

Chow dog was breathing better and was showing signs of annoyance with the endotracheal tube for he was chewing at it and salivating to a considerable degree. He could not swallow with the tube in place. Jo removed the tube and we carried our patient into critical care and placed him in a cage. I instructed Jo to keep a close eye on him while Marna and I walked down the street to have lunch together. Jo would call us there if any significant changes or if the owner phoned or came in. Marna and I ate a hurried lunch but enjoyed spending that limited time together. Jo never called and when we returned to the hospital, our patient was responding more to what was going on around him.

Chow dog was no longer on his side but resting on his sternum. His eyes were responding slightly to light but would not restrict completely. He was no longer drooling saliva and was able to swallow. He was in a semi-alert phase but completely confused as to where he was. The cage was new, he did not recognize our voices, and the odor of the zephrine on his scalp was a new smell he could not identify.

We monitored Chow dog all afternoon and when we got ready to leave, he was sitting up. A pan of water was placed in his cage and he tried to drink some but was unsteady when he crawled over to take a lap or two.

It was well past normal closing time and we still had not heard from the owner. I asked Jo to call the local newspaper and tell them that a black Chow was injured and hospitalized at our location. If anyone was planning to place an advertisement for a lost dog, this might help the owner locate their pet.

Later that night I had a call from a Long Beach hospital. Their answering service could not locate a veterinarian to take the emergency so the call was extended through the San Pedro hospital's exchange. I was now patched through the two answering services and talking to a Mr. Lester. He had a dog that was badly cut up and needed medical attention as soon as possible. I explained that I could not meet him at the Long Beach hospital for I had not contracted with that hospital for emergencies and did not have keys to get in. I would meet him at the San Pedro hospital if that was alright with him. "Look, doc. I will meet you anywhere!" I gave him instructions and was out the door.

Twenty minutes later I pulled into the hospital's parking lot and right behind me a station wagon with three adults arrived. One was driving and two were holding an English Setter wrapped in several bed sheets on their laps. Blood was oozing through the saturated sheet. I opened the door and they carried the injured dog into the treatment room as I had requested.

I sedated Cado and started an intravenous drip using a plasma expander. I hurriedly went to my car and retrieved the gas anesthetic machine, intubated Cado, and connected him to the gas. Next, I carefully rolled back the sheet and found that a tourniquet had already been put on his left front leg. Cado had cut himself when he went through a plate glass window. A deep cut was evident on his chest and several shards of glass sparkled over his body where they were held in place by dried blood.

I suggested that the Lesters leave Cado with me. They decided to go over to a nearby restaurant for a sandwich and coffee and would be back in about an hour.

I released the tourniquet and was able to locate the problem vessels and immediately tied them off. Next I checked the long gash on his chest and cauterized several small bleeders. I made a cursory exam over the rest of his body and found many lesions that needed my attention but I wanted to focus on the principal ones first—the leg and the chest. It took numerous sutures to close both of these major lacerations. I then got a pan of water and began giving him a "cat bath" one leg at a time, then one part of his body. I turned him over and checked his other side and proceeded in the same manner as before. Soon the sparkle from the glass was no longer evident and I had decided that surgery was completed.

Each of the minor cuts had been cleaned, derided, cauterized, and sutured as I went along. Cado certainly looked battle scarred for his hair had been clipped off wherever surgery was required. There were eight to ten minor locations where suturing had been a necessity. The plasma expander container was now empty and I switched to an intravenous drip of 5 percent saline and dextrose at one drop every six seconds. I administered antibiotics both intravenously and intramuscularly to protect him from infection.

I had been at work almost two hours. The men had returned from the restaurant and were sitting in their car waiting. They saw me unlock the front door and I beckoned for them to come in. While they watched Cado, I prepared a padded cage for his occupancy. Then they helped me place Cado in an intensive care cage with the drip still attached and running.

I had not taken time to fill out the patient/client history card so we went out in front to perform that task. Mr. Lester introduced me to his brother and his next door neighbor.

"What in the world happened?" I asked.

"Cado watches all of the neighborhood cats. He will run from one window to another in the house just to keep track of them as they journey around the house. He had been watching a cat from the bedroom window and I guess when the cat decided to run around the house, Cado ran to the living room and jumped up on the couch for better vision. The couch tipped over and broke the plate glass window behind it. The momentum catapulted Cado and most of the couch through the window. It made one heck of a noise and a huge mess."

Mr. Lester continued by saying, "I checked Cado immediately and called you. My brother applied the tourniquet and my neighbor came over to help. The back of the couch was cut up badly and will likely have to be reupholstered. We tilted the couch back into the living room and then headed here. The ladies said that they would clean up the living room."

The necessary deposit was left and Mr. Lester would call the hospital in the morning. I recommended a complete medicated bath prior to discharge to remove any unnoticed specks of glass as well as any blood stains on Cado's coat. Before they left, I showed them the pan that I had used to wash the lesions. In the bottom was about a teaspoon of fine glass that at one time had decorated Cado's blood-matted coat.

When I arrived at my office the following morning there was a camper parked on the street in front of my hospital. It had a Colorado license plate. As I approached the office door, a man got out and walked over to join me. He introduced himself as Walt Klosterman and asked me if by any chance I might have an injured Chow dog under my care. I said, "Yes, a black one." "That's probably Boris." He then walked over to his camper and told his wife that he thought that he had located Boris. I unlocked the door and we went inside. We could hear Boris whine even before we got back to the ward area for he had already recognized his master's voice and was eagerly waiting with his nose stuck between the cage bars and tail wagging.

Mrs. Klosterman said, "We had been visiting friends and had gone to Disneyland for an outing. Boris was left in the camper because his friends did not have a yard that would contain a dog. When we got back, the camper door was wide open and Boris was gone. Someone had broken into the camper but must have left in a hurry when they discovered a large Chow dog inside. Since the door was open, Boris decided to take a little walk and got out into the street traffic. Thank you so much for taking care of our precious pet."

# –17–

## A CANINE VISITOR

I was looking forward to the school's spring break with mixed emotions. When children are home for that week, gates and doors are accidentally left open and pets get into all sorts of problems. Accident cases, fight wounds, and foxtail abscesses are just a few of the circumstances that result when animals are allowed to roam. This means that I am more involved with emergencies when school is not in session and have less time to be home with Marna and the boys during that period of time.

There is, however, a positive aspect of having the boys at home. Allen and George both like to work at my hospital, so they usually work alternate days. This provides me with additional help and enables them to earn some extra spending money. Throughout the day we chat during the quieter moments and then we go out to lunch together if the situation permits.

When Allen and I arrived at my hospital, Mrs. Gibson was waiting with Mattie, a mixed Cocker breed. Mattie is an outside dog and roams their yard day and night. She had a swollen foot with an unsightly laceration completely around it.

Jo had already pulled the patient record card. I put on a smock and proceeded into the exam room with Mattie and Mrs. Gibson. Allen came in to help restrain Mattie while I surveyed the lesion. It was an unusual wound and I asked how it had happened. Mrs. Gibson said, "Mattie got tangled up in a loop of heavy duty twine that we use to hold up string beans. Apparently she could not get it off her foot so she just kept pulling at it and this action strangulated her paw and cut of the circulation. Her foot was badly swollen when I removed the twine. Doctor, do you think the accidental tourniquet was on so long that she might lose her foot?" It was a nasty wound and a wide one, too. The string had sawed through the skin and underlying tissue, reaching the bone in some places. Mrs. Gibson had to go to work so Mattie was left with us. She planned to phone later in the morning and see how her pet was doing.

Allen carried Mattie to the treatment room and I sedated her with some surital. The lesion was debrided and several sutures were taken. Fortunately the major vessels and nerves were still intact. The wound could not be closed in many places because there was over a half an inch gap where the string had sawed through the tissue. Several retention sutures were then used to keep the separated edges in close proximity.

The foot was then bandaged and placed into an aluminum walking splint for protection. It was imperative that Mattie could not gain access to the lesion and chew on it. The entire lower leg was wrapped in bandages and then secured with elastic tape. Antibiotics followed and Allen put Mattie with a plastic collar around her neck into a recovery cage that he had previously prepared.

Jo came back and told me that Pablo was visiting us again. Pablo lived about two blocks away and every time he got loose, he would come down to the hospital and visit us. If we were closed, he would lie down by the front door and wait. Pablo was a male German Shepherd who weighed about eighty pounds. Clients were very wary of him and would avoid him if possible, but it was hard to sidestep him when he was waiting at the hospital's front door.

In order to keep the normal traffic into the hospital it was necessary to bring Pablo inside and situate him in a cage. I located a leash and escorted Pablo to the rear of the hospital and asked Jo to call his owners and let them know where he was. Soon one of the Webster boys arrived to escort Pablo home.

Young Webster said, "I got into trouble for not latching the gate!" I explained to several clients that were in the reception room what Pablo did whenever he got loose. One of them remarked, "The last place I would camp on my day off would be at my doctor's office."

While I was discussing a case in the exam room with one of my clients, a lady brought in a full bucket of canine feces. She had called earlier about a worm problem that her St. Bernard may have and Jo had asked her to bring in a fecal sample for some laboratory work. Jo couldn't look at me when I stepped out of the exam room. She just showed me the bucket. I returned to the exam room for a tongue depressor and calmly took a fresh sample from the wide selection contained in the plastic bucket. I thanked the lady and told her that was all I needed. I took the sample into the lab. Jo was waiting for me there. She was laughing and holding her sides. I said, "Jo, she's all yours now!" Jo returned to the reception room and collected the laboratory fee.

The lady said, "Is that all the doctor needs?"

"Yes," was Jo's response, "You can take the rest home."

"But I am on my way to work."

Jo politely said, "We can dispose of it for you."

"You can keep that old bucket too!"

"We will do that also. Call us in a couple of hours for the lab results."

Jo came walking back to the rear of the hospital lugging a bucket of "you know what." All of us had a good laugh. Jo said, "I am never going to request a stool sample in the future without specifying the small quantity we need for analysis." The incident added considerable humor to our morning. When Allen and I drove home at day's end, he insisted that he be allowed to tell his mother first about the bucket incident.

I was sitting in my chair visiting with Marna and expecting the phone to ring at any time. It did. The Hawthorne operator had a Mrs. Nicholson on the line concerning their blond Cocker Spaniel, Vana, who had been loosing a lot of weight even though she had been eating all of the food that was offered to her. Mrs. Nicholson would appreciate it if I would see Vana this evening. I agreed to meet her at Hawthorne in a half an hour. Marna had just finished brewing a pot of coffee so she filled a styrofoam cup and handed it to me as I headed for my Mustang.

The entire Nicholson family was waiting for me when I arrived. I filled out the client/patient card and suggested that the three children wait in the reception room for it would be too crowded if all entered the exam room while I attended Vana. Mr. Nicholson placed Vana on the exam table and held her so she would not jump off. Her temperature was normal. I turned her around and got a whiff of a very ketotic breath. I then commenced my questioning.

"Does Vana eat all her food?"

"Yes, almost all that is offered to her."

"Does she drink a lot of water?"

"Yes, and that causes her to urinate a lot too."

"She seems to have lost considerable weight."

"I think that she has been losing weight for several weeks."

Mrs. Nicholson interrupted by saying, "Maybe the weight loss has been going on for several months."

There was an indication of considerable glucose in the urine sample. I returned to the front room, pulled up a chair and discussed my findings with the entire family.

"I believe that Vana has diabetes mellitus."

"That doesn't sound good, doctor."

"No, it doesn't. I would like to hospitalize Vana overnight and have this hospital run some more tests on the urine as well as the blood. I think that a second opinion is necessary. Would that be alright with you?"

"Yes, but if it means that we may have to give those insulin injections daily, I believe that we will have her put to sleep."

At this stage, the two older children understood what their father was saying and started crying. Two days later I had a phone call from the Hawthorne doctor. He informed me that Vana did have diabetes mellitus and he had just euthanized her. He thanked me for taking the case and was very sorry it turned out as it did. I thanked him for informing me and told him that I always appreciate a follow-up report on the emergencies I take for it helps me to become more astute in the way I handle emergency cases.

# -18-

# A STRANGE FELINE

**W**hen I walked in the door, I knew that I wouldn't be home long. Marna had four places set at the kitchen table and a brown bag was on the counter. Marna said that the San Pedro exchange had called and that the client was already on the way to that hospital. I exchanged my coat and tie for a sweater, picked up my sack dinner, and headed for the Mustang. I should have kept the motor running.

I pulled into the parking lot and the client was holding a Schipperke, one of those Dutch barge dogs, and was impatiently pacing back and forth in front of the hospital door. As I unlocked the hospital door, Mrs. Quincy said that Trailer had been badly burned. We went into the exam room and I checked Trailer's back. A large beet red area a little larger than my hand was evident between his shoulder blades.

I needed to know what kind of burn Trailer had received. As I looked up at Mrs. Quincy, she anticipated my question and said it was a hot water scald. Mrs. Quincy had been canning some fruit and had boiled water in order to sterilize the jar she was planning to use. "As I was moving the pan of hot water from one burner to another, I stepped back on Trailer's foot. He cried. I jumped and accidentally sloshed some of the hot water on him. Is he badly burnt, doctor?"

"I don't know yet," was my response.

I clipped the fur over the irritated area of Trailer's back and then rubbed in a liberal amount of furacin ointment. I crisscrossed a bandage

78

over his back and on each side of his front legs to help keep the bandage in place. I wanted the bandage to protect the wound if he began to pay attention to the irritating burn. The bandage would also hinder him if he decided to try and lick off the ointment.

I stepped into the pharmacy and made up a prescription of a mild tranquilizer in case his lesion began to annoy him. At the last moment, I dispensed some of the salve and a roller bandage with some adhesive tape. I explained that nothing needed to be done at home unless the bandage slipped out of position. An appointment was made for two days hence.

"Where did he get the name 'Trailer'?" I asked.

"He follows me around the house wherever I go. Sometimes he is so close that he almost touches me when I walk—more or less like a trailer would follow a car. When I stop, he stops. It is like we were connected with an invisible trailer hitch!"

I was chatting with Mrs. Quincy about some of Trailer's habits when the phone rang. It was the back line so I picked up the receiver. Marna had told the Hawthorne exchange that I was at the San Pedro hospital. A Mr. Gray was on the line. The operator said, "I don't understand his problem. Would you like to be connected?" I said that I would talk with him. Soon Mr. Gray was on the line. I waved to Mrs. Quincy as she departed with Trailer. Mr. Gray had an unusual problem. "When I got home from work and pulled into my garage, a strange animal, a cat I think, headed for cover under my work bench. It was not an ordinary cat in any sorts for it was spotted in color and had a longer tail than a domestic cat. I backed my car out into the driveway and closed the garage door—then I called the hospital."

"Did you also call the humane society?" I asked.

"No," he said, "If it is a wild animal of some kind, I didn't want them to have to kill it."

"Give me your address and I will be right over."

I finally located the street he was on in the Palos Verdes hills and was looking for his house number painted on the curb when I saw him wave from down the block. I pulled into his driveway and parked near his car. We went into the garage closing the door quickly behind us. He pointed to the far corner of the garage where the animal had sought refuge. Several boxes were piled there along with some firewood. The boxes were carefully removed and then slowly pieces of firewood were lifted off the pile. It was getting dark so Mr. Gray returned to the house and emerged with a flashlight. Two more pieces of wood were removed and we now had a glimpse of our intruder.

We did not have the necessary equipment to capture what appeared to be some sort of a member of the cat family, so I asked Mr. Gray to call the local humane society for a back up. I remained in the garage because if the animal knew someone was present, it would likely remain in what it thought would be a safe location.

About half an hour passed before the humane officer arrived. We agreed that we wanted to capture the animal without injuring it. Mr. Gray produced a large net that he used to put over his strawberry patch to keep the birds away and the officer brought in a large portable cage from his truck. We carefully covered the entire wood pile with the net and closed all the avenues of escape that we could perceive. Next we arranged the wood so that an escape tunnel was available. The next step was to get the animal to move and the best way was to frighten it into thinking that its present location was no longer a safe haven.

The opened cage was placed at the wood tunnel escape route and Mrs. Gray provided us with a couple of spoons and cookie sheets. We lowered the metal sheets as close to the intruder's location as possible then beat on them with the spoons. It worked. We now had a cat of some kind running into the cage. The cage door was quickly closed and latched and we had now trapped the mystery animal.

Mr. Gray asked, "What is it?" The humane officer had no idea. We did agree that it was a member of the feline family. Mrs. Gray now ventured out of the house with an camera and took several flash pictures. The officer left with the cat and said that he would take it to the Los Angeles Zoo in the morning.

The Grays invited me into the house and we opened the encyclopedia. We finally agreed that it was not a small ocelot but a margay—a South American member of the feline family. How it got into the Palos Verdes area was perplexing to all of us. We enjoyed a cup of coffee and a piece of pie and relived the evening's experience again. I was about to leave and head for home when I thought of calling Marna and checking in to see if any other calls were pending. She asked me to call the Lawndale exchange. I did and they gave me Mr. Pederson's number.

I called and Mr. Pederson said that when he got home from work and let the cat out of the house, he noticed that one of Mimic's eyes was almost closed and was noticeably tearing. He wanted to know where and when I could see Mimic. I agreed to meet him at the Lawndale hospital in twenty minutes.

Mr. Pederson arrived and seemed to be in quite a hurry. He wanted me to examine Mimic right away. I dropped some opthaine eye anesthetic into Mimic's right eye and then reflected the lower eyelid. It took only a moment to remove the foxtail. A floursescin strip test indicated that no corneal abrasion had occurred so I dispensed some cortisone eye ointment to be alternated every two hours with a gentocin durafilm solution.

As I was making out the charges and filling in the client/patient card, Mr. Pederson kept looking at his watch. Finally he broke the silence and said, "I am a pilot for Delta and just got in about seven and went home only to find Mimic in trouble. My wife is a flight attendant for the same airline and she arrives in about fifteen minutes and I promised to pick her up." I said, "You had better be on your way or both of us will be in trouble." I handed him the hospital's business card and asked him to call and report on Mimic's condition sometime the following afternoon. He bade me good-bye and hurried to his car.

I checked with Marna and no more calls were waiting so I headed home. I told the boys about the mysterious animal that the Grays had found in their garage and that I had no idea where it came from or to whom it belongs. Albert was sitting next to me and was very attentive and full of questions. I asked him to get the afghan blanket from our bedroom and I would show him what happened. We still had some logs on the hearth. I asked George to get Faux Pas's carrying cage. I placed the stuffed toy, Tigger, behind the woodpile and then threw the afghan over the pile carefully tucking the edges of it down so Tigger could not escape. Next I arranged the woodpile to leave an escape tunnel. Albert was asked to get a spoon and a pan. When all was ready, I asked him to beat on the pan. While Albert was beating and making all the noise and looking at his brothers for approval, I quickly grabbed Tigger, his favorite toy, and stuffed him into the cage. While doing this, I shouted, "We've got him, we've got him." George and Allen who had been watching their noise-making brother had not noticed what I had done and asked, "How did you get Tigger to go into the cage?"

Marna laughed at the charade and notified the rest of us that it was time for dessert. Moments later we were all eating strawberry shortcake.

The boys were busy on the couch asking each other how Tigger really got into the cage.

It had been a long day at my hospital and I had already responded to three emergencies that night. I was tired and sleeping soundly when the phone rang. The Torrance exchange had an emergency for me. I glanced at the clock and it was three in the morning. I dressed and left. I opened up the door and turned on the lights and waited for the client. Thirty minutes later I was still waiting and it was ten minutes to four.

At five after four, I called the Torrance exchange and asked them what happened to my client. They did not know. They hadn't called me. I called home. Marna said that the Palos Verdes operator wondered where I was and that the client was waiting there. I guess that I had been so tired that I had not listened carefully when the phone rang at three. I now realized that I had gone to the wrong hospital. I called the Palos Verdes service and told them if the client called back that I was only ten minutes away.

I arrived and faced an angry client by the name of Friedman. I tried to explain why I was late but it did little good. I located their card in the files and went into the exam room and looked at Tuffy. Tuffy was an Australian Shepherd and had a badly swollen ear. Mr. Friedman had let him out in the front yard to do his chores and a strange dog was around. A fight ensued and Tuffy had his ear bitten. His ear was now full of blood and standing out laterally. His ear bothered him and he showed his annoyance by periodically shaking his head.

Mr. Freidman had calmed down some by now and that enabled me to converse with him more easily. Tuffy would have to be put under anesthetic so his ear could be lanced and cared for. He agreed to leave Tuffy and call later in the morning. I again apologized for being late and he departed.

It was more of a puncture wound than a laceration. Undoubtedly the other dog's tooth had penetrated a blood vessel causing considerable hemorrhaging under the skin of the ear forming a huge pocket of blood. I lanced the ear and expelled the blood. It would only refill again unless I compressed the pocket where the blood had been. I located the button box that most veterinarians keep handy and selected eight buttons. Tuffy was put under anesthetic and connected to the metafane gas. I then used a button-like compress. A button was placed on each side of the ear and sutured together through the button holes then snugged down against the skin to close the potential blood pocket. This was repeated three more times until all four button compresses were completed to my satisfaction.

Tuffy was put into a recovery cage, I cleaned up the surgical mess, and returned my anesthetic machine out to my car before I headed for home. No lights were on when I pulled into the driveway but when I got into the house, Marna was meandering down the hall in robe and slippers.

The next morning I had showered and freshened up and by the time I got out into the kitchen the boys were waking up. Marna poured me a cup of coffee to go with the stack of buckwheat pancakes that she had so graciously prepared. I almost fell asleep at the kitchen table. Allen had to be at school early so I dropped him off on my way to the office. Another day lay ahead of me.

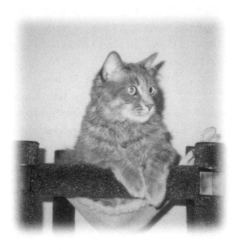

# -19-

## Horse Work

**W**e had just eaten dinner on Friday evening and I sat down in the family room to go through the day's mail when the phone next to me rang. It was the exchange of Dr. Jackson, an equine practitioner, wanting to know if I would speak to a client of his about an injured horse. I had not treated a horse since I had graduated from veterinary school, and I relayed this to the operator. She informed me that Dr. Jackson was out of town and the person filling in for him could not be reached. "It sounds to me like a real emergency. Would you at least talk to Mr. Martin and give him some advice?" I agreed to listen to what he had to say and was connected immediately.

The Martins had a horse that was breathing with considerable difficulty because of a neck injury. "Thanks for taking the call, doc," was the first comment I heard. "I know that you are a small animal vet but I need some advice. My mare was being chased by a dog and was frightened. She ran into a pipe fence in her paddock and fell down. When she got to her feet, she just stood there quietly, and is now breathing with difficulty. Jackson's exchange contacted several small animal vets but they wouldn't even talk to me. I can hear her breathing twenty feet away. I don't know what to do. Can you give me any advice?"

I got his address and told him that I would be there as soon as I stopped at my hospital for some supplies and equipment. "Hurry, doc, I don't want to lose my mare!" were Mr. Martin's last words before I hung up. I stopped by my hospital and picked up the two largest endotracheal tubes that had inflatable cuffs on them, grabbed a surgical pack, scalpel blades, gauze, gloves, and tape. I put them into a cardboard box, looked at the instructions that I had written down, and headed for Rolling Hills.

I pulled into the driveway and Mr. Martin met me and took me out to the corral where his Arabian mare was standing with her neck stretched out. Noisy sounds were coming from her whenever she inhaled or exhaled. I asked him to get a bucket of warm water and then cross-tie the mare in its stall. I felt the trachea and there was a definite indentation in the tracheal rings at about the same height as the top pipe in the corral fence. I scrubbed the neck down and prepared for surgery.

The surgical pack was opened and I put a blade on the scalpel handle then made a vertical incision over the trachea just dorsal to the injury. The sterno-hyoidial muscles were exposed and separated. This exposed the trachea to full view. A small incision was made between the tracheal rings and the largest tracheal tube was inserted. The mare started breathing better right away. I inflated the cuff and clamped off the small rubber tube to the cuff. Both Mr. Martin and I gave a sigh of relief.

Elastic tape was put around the horse's neck and the tracheal tube was taped to it to stabilize the tube's position. I asked Mr. Martin to find a rubber band for me. When he had returned, I placed a thin layer of gauze over the exposed end of the tracheal tube and secured it with the rubber band. This would insure that no dust or chaff would be inhaled and cause an inhalation pneumonia

I said, "Call me if your mare has any trouble. Leave her cross-tied so she will not rub the tube out of position and have Dr. Jackson check her as soon as possible."

He went to the house and brought out another bucket of warm water and a bar of soap. I cleaned up my hands and arms and then looked at the front of me. I did not have the luxury of owning any coveralls that large animal veterinarians use and blood had stained my clothes from my chest to my shoes.

He got out his check book to take care of the account but I said that I didn't know what the charges would be. "I'll let Dr. Jackson bill you and then he can square up with me." Mrs. Martin arrived with two mugs of coffee and we visited for fifteen minutes or so before I left for home.

The next day was Saturday and I had another call concerning an injured horse. Dr. Jackson was still out of town. His answering service said,

"Hi, its me again!" I said, "Who's me?" She laughed and said, "Dr. Jackson's exchange. I have another injured horse for you. The owner, Miss McFarland, has called. Will you talk to her?" I asked her to connect me for I felt that no harm could be done if I only had to talk with the owner.

Miss McFarland was on the line and her horse had injured itself under its jaw and was bleeding badly. She said that the blood was spurting and that indicated to me the likelihood of arterial bleeding. I told her that I would be on my way as soon as I stopped at my hospital. I picked up the supplies that I felt I needed and, with the direction diagram beside me, I again returned to the Rolling Hills area. I had remembered seeing the road name some months ago. Only three homes were on it so in no time I was unpacking my gear and walking toward the horse barn.

Both Mr. McFarland and his daughter, Lisa, greeted me and ushered me into Poco's stall. Poco was flaying her head around and blood was being thrown in all directions. There was no way that I could inspect the wound unless Poco's head could be held still. Mr. McFarland tried to ear the mare down [restrain the horse by pulling down an ear] but that only helped a little. He asked Lisa to get the twitch and when that was applied to Poco's upper lip, she stood stock still.

Using gauze sponges, I packed the area and soon located the mandibular artery that was causing the problem. It had been severed so I clamped it off with forceps and then ligated it. A few other collateral vessels that had been bleeding were pressure packed with gauze that Lisa held in place. It was a nasty looking skin lesion. It almost looked like a triangle or maybe "T" shaped. I trimmed up the edges by debriding the tissue and then put in several sutures to unite the opposing edges. When I finished, it looked as if I may have used a darning technique.

I asked how it happened and they did not know. Lisa had come out to feed Poco and the top board on the fence had blood on it. Several other spots around the paddock were decorated in blood also. Since Poco had been in the paddock all of the time, we decided to walk the premises and see what we could find. Mr. McFarland made the initial discovery. A metal fence post in line with the corral fence was sticking up maybe six inches higher than the top rail and had blood and horse hair on it. Poco had likely raised her head high enough and then brought it down on the post. The post had acted like a spear and punctured a hole between Poco's left and right mandibular bones causing the lesion. The mystery case had now been solved.

We all went into the tack room where there was a sink and washed up. I was bloody to my elbows where blood had run down my arms. All of us were spotted with drops of blood. I suggested cross-tying Poco for two or three days or until Dr. Jackson decided otherwise.

"Let me step into the house for my checkbook," said Mr. McFarland. I suggested, as I had with Mr. Martin, that it would be better if Dr. Jackson sent him a bill since I was not familiar with large animal fees. I suggested that they wash Poco down and clean up the blood to avoid a fly problem. They thanked me and I left for home.

Dr. Jackson called me two days later and thanked me for assisting him in taking care of his clients. He said that he had gone to an equine symposium out of state for four days and the person who was covering for him was inundated with work because so many of the equine practitioners from this area had attended the conference. I told Dr. Jackson that I had left the charges up to him because I did not know the mileage or stop fees. I did tell him how long I was at each location. He said that he would put my check in the mail immediately. I explained what I had done and asked him to check them out soon because he may be able to give the owners better advice.

"Let's get together for lunch sometime next week when I get caught up on my back load of cases," Dr. Jackson said.

"Call me whenever," was my reply.

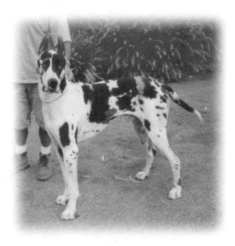

# —20—

# THE TREE HOUSE

**I**t was a warm evening and all of us were out on the patio enjoying a cool drink and planning what we were going to do the coming holiday weekend. The boys finally agreed unanimously to go to the beach. Marna said she would take them Saturday morning while I was at the office. I could not go anyway since I would be out of telephone range.

We were deciding what food to take on the forthcoming picnic when the phone rang. The Manhattan Beach hospital had a Mr. Turner on the line. His dog had just fallen out of a tree. "Mac is injured and needs to be seen soon." "How long will it take you to get to the hospital?" I asked. "Less than fifteen minutes," was Mr. Turner's response. "You may have to wait a few minutes for me. I plan to leave immediately." I headed for my Mustang.

Mr. Turner was there with his ten-year-old son when I arrived. Mac was carried directly into the treatment room. I established a bottle of 5 percent saline and dextrose immediately when I saw how pale he was and then added solu-delta-cortef to it to counteract the shock that was exhibited. I palpated Mac's abdominal cavity and could feel solution sloshing around. I tapped the abdomen with a large needle and extracted frank blood. I immediately established another intravenous drip with a plasma expander.

I pondered the idea of taking Mac directly into surgery for I suspected the possibility of a ruptured spleen. I prepared surgery for this possibility and then decided to go ahead and implement what my intuition felt was likely. Mac was scrubbed down, prepped, and draped. A ventral midline incision was made and blood immediately appeared. I packed off the area and commenced searching for the cause of the internal hemorrhaging. The spleen was exposed and it had ruptured. Next I double clamped all of the vessels leading to the spleen and cut between the clamps. The spleen was removed from the body and all of the incoming arteries were ligated. Then the clamps on each were removed. I carefully searched for other possibilities of hemorrhaging but found none. Abdominal closure was completed. I checked the refrigerator and found a unit of canine blood and connected it with the drip line that once was used for the plasma expander.

Mac was still out of it but his mucous membranes were gradually turning from a grayish color to a healthy pink. I monitored Mac carefully while I cleaned up the surgery room. He was gradually improving. The surgery was still a mess and I felt that it would be poor judgement to have the Turners come in and visit Mac when there was a bloody mess. I prepared a cage in critical care and carefully moved Mac into a clean area with the two drip lines still connected. I washed up and changed into a smock and went out to talk to the anxious Turners who had been waiting patiently.

Mr. Turner had his arm around his son and was reassuring him that Mac would be fine. They both looked up when I entered. I told them that I had done a splenectomy and I felt that Mac would be up and around in a few days. Tears of joy filled the young lad's eyes.

I said, "If I heard you correctly when you first came in, you told me that Mac fell out of a tree." Mr. Turner looked at his son and said, "Tell the doctor what happened. Tell him how Mac got up in the tree." The youngster started talking very softly and was holding his head down as if he was speaking to the floor. "Well, Dad said not to take Mac up to my tree house, but I didn't mind. I made a container and put Mac in it and then attached a rope and pulled him up to the house. When he got up, I let him out of the box. He was very scared. I turned around to do something and when I looked back, Mac was hanging on to the edge of the floor with his front feet. Before I could reach him, he fell." Mr. Turner added, "He must have fallen eighteen to twenty feet."

The lad continued, "Mac sounded like a pumpkin when he hit the ground. He did not move and I thought that he was dead. I ran inside and got Dad." I looked up at Mr. Turner and said, "I don't think your son will take Mac up to the tree house again. I think that he has learned his lesson, don't you?" Mr. Turner agreed and said, "There is no better teacher than experience." The three of us went next door to get something to drink. When we left, the young man came over and thanked me with a hug and promised to listen to his father's wisdom in the future.

When we returned to the hospital, I felt that it was time for Mac to have some visitors. Mac was not standing up yet, but he had rolled over on his chest. The transfusion had been completed and I disconnected it. The dextrose and saline drip tubing had been chewed into and the remaining solution had soaked into the towels that Mac was lying on. With Mr. Turner and his son helping, we moved Mac to a clean, dry cage and put on another unit of saline and dextrose. I administered it at a rate of one drop every six seconds. The Turners administered a loving pat to their pet and friend, and we all headed for our individual homes.

I responded to several emergencies during the early afternoon and evening. It was four o'clock in the morning when I awoke and grabbed the phone before it woke up the entire family. The Palos Verdes operator had a Mrs. Bosworth on the line concerning a vomiting dog. I asked to be connected to the distressed client.

"This is the doctor speaking. May I help you?"

"Yes, doctor, My dog chewed up a guest's fur coat earlier in the evening and he started vomiting about an hour ago and it hasn't let up since."

"Has he vomited up anything yet or has he had just dry heaves?"

"Only a bit of fluid. But he definitely has the heaves. Here, I will hold my phone down near him and you can hear what he is doing."

I could easily hear a dog retching in the background but now it was much more pronounced with the phone near the dog's head.

"I think that it would be wise if I saw him. Can you meet me at the hospital in thirty minutes?"

"I'll be there," was Mrs. Bosworth's response.

I arrived within thirty minutes and had to wait another half an hour for the client to arrive. I was about to phone the operator when the Bosworth car pulled into the parking lot. Mrs. Bosworth apologized for being late and remarked that her husband insisted on putting several blankets on the backseat of their Mercedes in case Ike puked in the car. Mrs. Bosworth brought Ike into the hospital. He had stopped once in the parking lot and again in the reception room to disgorge foamy sputum. Ike was a male chocolate Labrador and weighed approximately sixty pounds.

"You aren't my regular doctor."

"No, I only take emergencies for this hospital."

"Would you call my regular doctor immediately!"

"He's not available tonight and I am responding to his calls."

"Well, I guess that you will have to do!"

I picked up Ike and placed him on the exam table. He tried to vomit again but all that was emitted was foam.

"You mentioned on the phone that he had chewed up a fur coat. Is that correct?"

"Yes. We had a dinner party at our house for the Democratic Fund Raising Committee. The ladies put their furs and other wraps on the bed upstairs. Ike pulled one of the coats off the bed and dragged it to the corner of the room and proceeded to chew it up. He destroyed it beyond repair. It was embarrassing—it was a very expensive coat. When the guests found out what Ike had done, they teased the owner of the coat by saying that only Ike would have known that it was a rabbit fur. This added to our embarrassment. However, the owners were very nice and reassured us by saying that the coat was fully insured."

I rationalized that the fur had formed a mass in Ike's stomach similar to a hair ball in a cat. It needed some kind of lubrication to pass out of the stomach either one way or the other. I located a stomach tube and pumped in a couple ounces of mineral oil into my patient and then put him into a run while both Mrs. Bosworth and I waited for results.

I asked Mrs. Bosworth if she would like a cup of coffee. She said, "Yes, if it is real coffee." I then fixed her what she had requested and joined her with my own cup of decaffeinated coffee.

I checked on Ike fifteen minutes later and he had expelled a couple of mats of hair—one had a button in it. He was feeling much better as time went on. I suggested to Mrs. Bosworth that she might as well go home because Ike might vomit some of the oily hair mats all over their nice car. I said that I would call her later in the morning when I stopped by to check on Ike on the way to my own practice.

"You mean that you are not going to remain here with my dog?"

"Yes, Ike will be fine but just needs to have time to rid himself of all that fur he ingested."

"Listen, doctor, I insist that you stay with Ike in case he needs more help."

I agreed to Mrs. Bosworth's request and dog-sat my patient for the remainder of the morning until the regular veterinarian arrived to take over. Ike vomited a little more fur and then passed an oil soaked stool that contained another button. When the staff arrived, Ike was prancing around his cage and ready to go home.

I called Marna and asked her to bring my shaving kit to my office so I could make myself more presentable to my own clients. Jo arrived at the hospital first and commented about my bedraggled appearance. I only shrugged and said that I would explain what happened later. In the meantime Marna had dropped off my shaving gear. Soon I was refreshed and fully awake to take on the challenges of a new day.

Jack, my colleague from the Palos Verdes hospital, called about ten that morning. He said that Mrs. Bosworth was pleased that Ike was doing well. "She is rather demanding and insisted that we have Ike bathed and ready to go home at nine this morning. However, she did remark that she insisted that you stay and keep an eye on Ike until I arrived. I charged out your extra time and she paid the bill without batting an eye. I'll drop your fee in today's mail."

It was still light outside when my first call came in that evening. It was from the answering service at my own hospital in Redondo Beach. Mrs. Nuñez had a cat that had an injured foot and wondered if I could see it this evening. She apologized for disturbing me at home but she was very concerned about Carter. I agreed to meet her in twenty minutes.

George went with me and we arrived at the same time as our client. Mrs. Nuñez had walked as she lived nearby and had Carter in a cardboard box in a shopping cart. My son got out a blank patient card and I filled it out in the exam room. Carter was or had been a feral [wild] cat that had been domesticated. He was a shorthair yellow cat with a wonderful temperament indicating he had received a lot of love and kindness.

Carter's front left foot was bleeding and blood spots on the exam table were noted. Carter obviously preferred that I did not touch his foot so George brought in a blanket from the back of the hospital. We rolled Carter up in the blanket and then carefully extracted the injured paw for better scrutiny.

Mrs. Nuñez informed me what had happened. "Carter was a wild cat that I adopted. He comes into the house to eat because if I leave food outside all of the homeless cats eat the food. I also own a parrot. Carter watches the parrot and he sometimes jumps from the table to bat at the parrot's cage that is about as high as my head. This causes the parrot to squawk and that just excites Carter, and he will try it again and again. I think he used to survive on the birds he could catch before I started feeding him."

George held the blanket roll snugly and I examined the extended foot. Two nails were broken off and one of them had broken off so deeply that it was bleeding.

"Did Carter ever catch his claws on the bird cage?" I asked.

"Oh, yes, sometimes he would hang on to the cage for a moment or two swinging back and forth."

"What would your parrot do then?"

"Sometimes he would peck at Carter's feet but most of the time he would just ruffle up his feathers and squawk."

"Between the possibility of your parrot biting Carter or Carter hooking his nails on the cage—either situation could have caused the injury."

I trimmed all of his nails before bandaging the injured foot. I then gave him an antibiotic injection of penicillin to deter the possibilities of an infection. I put Carter in the box and the box in the grocery cart. I handed George the patient card to take care of the financial part of the evening while I cleaned up the exam room.

Moments later George stepped back into the exam room and quietly informed me that Mrs. Nuñez had no money. I stepped out to the front desk and Mrs. Nuñez immediately apologized about having me come out at night when she knew that she could not pay for my services. "Doctor, when Carter started tracking blood across the floor, I was worried and needed your help."

I assured her that there would be no charges for the emergency care of her pet. She thanked me and said that she would pay me as she could. I explained to her that there were no charges at all. She again thanked me. George came out of the back of the hospital with a ten pound bag of dry cat food that was a sample bag from a vender. He put it into the shopping cart next to Carter's box and helped guide Mrs. Nuñez through the front door. Mrs. Nuñez thanked us again. She said, "My friends sometimes call me Carter because I push this cart around and collect things. I thought that would be a good name for my cat, too."

# —21—

## NO DRY EYES

I had received a call through my own hospital exchange from the Eardleys. Now that I was also taking some emergency calls from my own hospital, I had a distinct advantage because I was usually acquainted with both the client and the patient. This was not the case at the other hospitals that I had contracted with for emergency coverage.

The Eardleys wanted to meet me at my hospital in Redondo Beach to see Gringo, an aged Labrador Retriever mix, that they wanted me to put to sleep. Gringo had experienced seventeen summers and his health had deteriorated to such a degree that his quality of life was questioned. During this past Easter vacation, the Eardleys and their children—two sons and a daughter—had mutually agreed that Gringo was suffering. That was two months ago and the situation had grown worse.

I pulled into the parking lot and before I had a chance to exit my car, the Eardleys arrived. They all wanted to be together as a family when Gringo breathed his last breath.

The necessary papers were completed and signed. The exam room was slightly crowded and I filled a syringe as all stood there quietly while their oldest son held Gringo. I located a vein and slowly administered the solution as Gringo settled gently into his arms and breathed his last gasp before he relaxed completely.

There was not a dry eye in the entire room and that included mine. Each member of the family patted their canine friend and gave him a hug for the last time. Mom and the three children beat a hasty tear-filled retreat to their car. Mr. Eardley visited with me a minute or two while he wrote a check. He remarked that this was the last pet they would ever own. He said, "We just can't handle the stress of moments like this. You know Rob, my oldest son, and Gringo are the same age." Mr. Eardley thanked me and shook my hand then he, too, retreated to his car.

I watched him climb into his car and realized that I had not given him a poem that I had written that I frequently give to my clients when they are under this stressed condition. It is as follows:

Each life is touched by God's own hand—
The animals and birds that live this land.
They all have a certain time on earth
That interval life between death and birth.

God has granted them a special time
To stand beside of all mankind.
Of dogs, cats and pets I speak, you see
For they will not live as long as me.

If I had selected their life of time,
Their life would be as long as mine.
But He does not agree with me
It's His wisdom that directs eternity.

My pet is growing old, I know
And it will pass before I go.
I will grieve and I will fret
And of my pet I'll not forget.

Yet when the pangs of grief are gone
I'll go out and find another one.
I love each pet, may its life be free
Until God again takes my pet from me.

"Tad" 1968

About one in the morning, I responded to my third emergency of the night. The Fieldings had called the Lawndale hospital about Sassy, their cat, who they thought might have been hit by a car. The Fieldings lived much closer to the hospital than I and were waiting as I pulled into the parking lot. In a cardboard cat carrying case was Sassy, their Abyssinian cat. We went into treatment and I began my exam of the patient before me.

Sassy had fluid in her abdomen. Her claws, especially her front ones, were frayed. She had indeed been hit by a car. This was confirmed by the Fieldings who had been watching television and heard car brakes squeal. Mrs. Fielding said, "I looked out the window and saw a man looking around his car. He even looked under his car and then gave a perplexed shrug, got into his car and drove away. I think that it is likely he hit Sassy but she was strong enough to run back to our house. Ten minutes later she cried at the front door. My husband opened the door and she more or less staggered into the house, walked two or three feet, and then lay down on the carpet. This was not like her at all."

I palpated her abdomen but could not identify her bladder. I passed a urinary catheter and then attached a syringe and injected almost twenty milliliters of air through the catheter. I then took a lateral and dorso-ventral views of her abdomen on the X-ray machine. My intention was to delineate the bladder wall by means of a pneumocystogram. We looked at the wet radiograph together and no delineation of the bladder wall was noted. Air was now evident in the abdominal cavity. Sassy had a ruptured urinary bladder.

Sassy was weak now from the trauma and the release of blood and urine into the abdominal cavity. The Fieldings kept an eye on their cat while I ventured out to my car and brought in the anesthetic machine. I then passed a feline endotracheal tube and connected Sassy to the inhalant gas. The Fieldings went home and I went to work.

I started an intravenous drip and added solu-delta-cortef for shock. I slowed the flow down to one drop every four seconds before preparing her for surgery. I put a keeper suture on the urinary catheter to keep it in place for I did not want the bladder to refill and put any stress of the suture line of the bladder. The abdominal cavity was lavaged several times to remove any urine as well as blood that had collected from the torn bladder wall. Surgery was completed and I carried Sassy into the intensive care ward and situated her on several towels. I rechecked the intravenous flow and reduced it slightly.

Sassy was still under the effects of the anesthetic when I closed her cage door. I returned the anesthetic machine to my car and then went back into surgery and cleaned up. Instruments were scrubbed and incorporated into a pack and then sterilized in the autoclave. I did not wish to leave my patient until she showed some signs of waking up. Time was still on my hands so I made a cup of instant coffee before making the necessary entries on the client card. By this time Sassy was responding to the blink reflex when I touched her brow. The hospital now was as clean and orderly as when I arrived so I headed for the door and then home.

I didn't want to disturb Marna so I curled up on the couch in the family room. Marna awakened me with a gentle tap on my shoulder. It seemed that I had only been asleep for a few minutes when in reality I had slept a solid four hours. The boys were stirring and the aroma of coffee permeated the air. I decided to shower and shave. When I stepped out of the shower, I found a cup of hot coffee resting on the bathroom counter. I dressed and refilled my cup to take with me. I wanted to check on Sassy before I got to my own hospital to take care of my scheduled surgeries. Marna handed me two pieces of toast that surrounded a slice of ham as I was stepping out the back door. The ham sandwich and coffee occupied my time as I drove to Lawndale and then to my hospital in Redondo Beach.

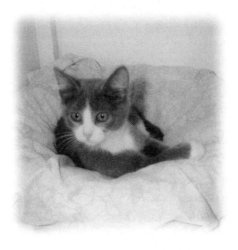

—————⋀————— **22** –

# A MIRROR IMAGE—ALMOST

**I**t was Monday morning. It had been a very busy weekend. I had responded to six emergencies on Saturday and I had seventeen cases on Sunday. I highlighted some of the cases for Jo and enjoyed a cup of coffee that she had just brewed at the same time. Somehow we got involved in a discussion of pet personalities.

We agreed that it was common to see a dog pulling an owner down the street toward the hospital and then when the owner turned toward our front door, the situation changed. The owner now had to drag her pet inside. It was exactly what happed ten minutes later. Mrs. Tovar dragged her Labrador Retriever, Ryan, through the front door of our hospital. Jo gave me a quick glance and then turned to locate the Tovar card. Ryan had been licking a spot on his back leg and it was now raw and moist, causing a lesion we call a hotspot.

Jo assisted me in lifting Ryan to the top of the exam table. It appeared to be a typical hot spot to my estimation. I clipped the area around the lesion until normal tissue was present. I then gently scrubbed the moist area with surgical soap and followed that by rubbing in a soothing vanishing cream base that contained an antibiotic and a steroid. Antibiotic and steroid injections followed. The same ointment was dispensed for Mrs. Tovar to administer to Ryan and instructions were given for his care.

I was standing behind the reception desk talking to a client when the Eardleys walked through the door at closing time. In their arms was a puppy that they had just acquired. It was uncommon for me to position myself behind the counter at this time of day because it interfered with Jo's job of closing the daily books. The Eardleys patiently waited for me to hang up the phone. Jo politely crowded me out of the way so she could complete her job and go home.

I had not seen the Eardleys since Gringo had died. Now they stood there holding a little pup that had many of Gringo's features. This was a surprise to me and totally unexpected for they had vowed to never own a pet again.

Mrs. Eardley held the adoption papers from the local humane society and presented them to me for the courtesy health examination. Jo searched the retired files for the Eardley card and presented that to me as well. Their daughter, Sue, had decided to come in as well so the three Eardleys, the puppy, and I went into the exam room. They had selected the name of Chum for their new arrival.

Chum was almost the same color pattern as Gringo, but where Gringo exhibited black spots, Chum was brown and where Gringo was brown, Chum was black. The reverse in the color pattern did remind me of Gringo and I could see why this pup caught their eye at the pound.

I had cautioned them that if they ever got another dog, they should never expect it to replace Gringo. Instead, it should have the opportunity to grow up with its own personality, quirks, and habits. Never, never try to force it into the mold of its predecessor. Already, however, they were comparing the two.

Sue was delighted to hold Chum. I carefully examined Chum and wrote down on the patient card his name, color, age, and gender. The temperature, pulse, and respiration were also recorded and his first distemper and parvovirus vaccines were given. Flea control, diet, and vitamin supplements were discussed and dispensed as needed. Sue then bundled him up and took him out to the car for his first visit to his new home.

Later that night I had a call from Mrs. Tovar through my hospital's exchange. Ryan was still chewing at the irritated portion of his skin and now a new spot was evident on his hip. Ryan's incessant chewing was driving her crazy. She had not given Ryan the medicated bath that I had recommended and wanted me to see Ryan again—right away. I met her at the hospital a little later and admitted Ryan. Both spots looked bad. I had no intention of giving Ryan a medicated bath that time of night so

I installed an Elizabethan plastic collar so he would be unable to reach the lesions in question. I told Mrs. Tovar that he would have the necessary medicated bath first thing in the morning when the kennel staff arrived.

I checked with Marna before I left and there were no further calls. Marna suggested that I pick up some dessert to share with the boys. I stopped and bought an apple pie and a quart of ice cream. Marna warmed up the pie and then converted it to pie á la mode with the addition of vanilla ice cream for all of us to enjoy.

The next morning the Eardleys were on the phone. Chum had cried all night. Advice was needed. The family had rotated the responsibility of holding Chum during his first night. When he was held, he would snuggle down in the holder's lap, stop crying, and go to sleep. The warmth of their human bodies was comforting and allowed him to doze off into the land of puppy slumber. Mr. Eardley realized that this dog-sitting routine could not go on forever and he needed some advice on how to alleviate the problem. I suggested using a ticking clock to simulate a mother's heartbeat and a hot water bottle or heating pad for warmth.

The next morning they were on the phone again. Jo handed me the phone and shrugged. The clock and heating pad system did not work. It appeared to them that Chum wanted company. They had a cat that slept with Gringo and I suggested they put Chum into the cat basket and see if that would quiet him during the night hours. After all, it was worth a try.

They phoned again the following morning. Their cat didn't mind the puppy except that the pup kept trying to nurse her. When this would happen, the cat would vacate the basket and perch on some high object out of Chum's reach. I began to think that my comments were becoming more of a sympathetic nature than a constructive nature. The end result was that Chum would visually locate the cat and then whine for it to come down from its protective position. The Eardley family was beginning to show signs of much needed sleep.

Mr. Eardley decided to help his family out on Friday night since he did not have to go to work the following day. His wife and daughter were in need of a good night's rest. The master of the house got up to puppy-sit when Chum cried. He poured himself a tot of brandy, turned on the television, and settled down for the rest of the night in his reclining chair with Chum cradled in his lap.

Mr. Eardley went to sleep and the brandy glass in his hand gradually slipped out of his grip and hit the floor. This awakened both dog and master. Mr. Eardley got up and went into the kitchen for paper towels to clean up the mess. When he returned, there was no brandy on the floor. Chum had taken care of that problem. He sat there smacking his lips and had a proud look on his face because he had helped. Chum slept well the rest of the night.

Mr. Eardley felt that if the late night toddy worked once, it might work again. It was three days before I was called. The family was getting a full night's sleep. Chum slept soundly also. When the Eardleys came in with Chum for his second vaccine, they said that they gradually reduced Chum's nightcap over about a week's interval and now he was on the wagon and doing well.

Chum continued to baffle the Eardleys. During the first week at home, he got into Sue's closet, rummaged around, and carried out one of Gringo's favorite toys. This old teddy bear had first belonged to their oldest son, Rob, and later claimed by Gringo. Now Chum had proclaimed possession of teddy. Teddy was now Chum's special treasure. He objected if the family took it from him. If the cat got too close to Teddy, Chum would growl. Teddy slept with Chum as it had with Gringo. Finally, the Eardley family was able to sleep well, too.

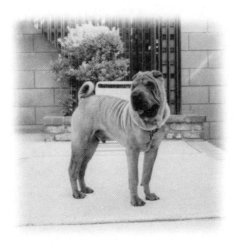

# –23–

## TABLE TALK

**M**arna had fixed a wonderful dinner and we were in our formal dining room. George had just completed thanking our Lord for His provision when the telephone rang. I answered the call from the hallway phone between the dining room and the kitchen. The operator had a client on the line that just wanted to ask me some questions. I obliged and was cross connected. The conversation involved a pet that had a parasite problem—namely a worm problem. I discussed the way the problem should be addressed—both what he should do by collecting a fecal sample and the choices that could be made depending on what the laboratory work revealed.

When I returned to the dining room, my three sons and Marna all had pale looks on their faces. Apparently my voice was so loud that they were able to hear my entire conversation with the client. I apologized for my lack of consideration and started to say more. Allen interrupted and said, "Don't even think about telling us about your phone conversation. Remember, Dad, that you are not supposed to talk about anything like that at the dinner table." I closed my mouth without saying another word. I looked around the table and each one sitting there gave me a glance of approval. I often needed to be reminded of this habit of mine.

After supper, I received a call from a Mrs. Prentice concerning her pet cat, Jester. I had remembered seeing Jester several months ago on an emergency but couldn't remember what the emergency was until she refreshed my memory. Mrs. Prentice greeted me with, "I am not happy about having to see you again but Jester has the same problem as she had before. She has been in a cat fight and has another abscess. I go to work early in the morning and would not be able to drop her off, so it would probably be best to have you see her tonight. Would that be possible?" I arranged to meet her at the Palos Verdes hospital in twenty minutes.

I looked at my watch as I pulled out of the garage. It was eight in the evening. I pointed my Mustang west toward the Pacific Ocean and headed toward the hospital that was only two blocks from the coastline. Mrs. Prentice was on time and I held the door open as she entered with a carrying cage that contained her pet. Jester was a calico, short-haired female about five years old. She had a very evident abscess on her right hip. It was going to be necessary to lance and drain the abscess and then place a seton as I had done before only this time it was in a different location.

Mrs. Prentice said, "I thought only male cats fought each other over the affections of a female. Jester seems to get into frequent squabbles so I have to confine her to the house. When I do this, she annihilates my upholstered furniture and drapes. I wish that I could stop that habit!"

"Maybe you should consider declawing her. This surgery would make it impossible for her to preen her front claws on the furniture."

"But if I put her outside she will not be able to defend herself!"

"Not necessarily. If she has weapons to fight with, like her claws, she will probably remain aggressive. If you remove the claws, many times a cat will become more passive and avoid fights."

"Maybe that is the thing to do. She averages about three abscesses a year and it is becoming rather expensive."

Jester had already been deposited into a cage in the treatment ward and I suggested that she have the surgery done the following morning by the regular hospital staff. The next day's staff would correct the abscess while Jester was under the same anesthetic. Mrs. Prentice hesitated for a few moments and then went along with what I had recommended. She added, "It will also save me the cost of hose since she destroys them also."

I asked her to call early the following morning after she had thought about my suggestion. This would give her a chance to confer with her regular doctor before they commenced administering the anesthetic. Mrs. Prentice said, "I really hate to do this!" I again assured her explaining that when you take a wild-natured animal and remove it from its natural environment, like inside a house, sometimes things have to be adjusted to make humans and cats compatible. Mrs. Prentice nodded in affirmation and left for home. I put water into Jester's cage and soon I was on my way also.

About midnight I was back at the same hospital looking at two male dogs that had been in a fight. Both pets belonged to the same owner. The Rottweiler was named Rhody and the Newfoundland's name was Fargo. Mrs. Curry was holding Fargo out in the reception room on a leash while I was scrutinizing Rhody who had been placed on the exam table by her husband. Mr. Curry was explaining to me that every time the dog two doors down the street came in heat, his two male dogs would get into an altercation. Rhody needed a few wounds sutured so we went into the treatment room and I used a cetacaine anesthetic spray to numb the tissue. I then placed two sutures into three separate lacerations. One other lesion required four sutures to completely close the wound. Now Rhody sported four spots that had been clipped and painted with red zephrine. Mr. Curry placed him on the floor, took him out to his wife, and returned with Fargo.

Fargo had gotten the best of the squabble except for a two-inch gash in his left ear that had gone completely through the cartilage of his right ear. It was necessary to sedate the Newfoundland with surital and put six to seven sutures on each side of the ear after first uniting the torn ear cartilage with four stainless steel sutures. The same antibiotic was given to prevent the numerous unseen tooth punctures wounds from becoming infected. The sedation did not last long and Fargo was almost fully awake as I completed the final suture. I then placed Fargo on the floor and escorted him to the front room. He was slightly unsteady on his feet but managed to walk without any assistance.

Mrs. Curry asked me if this routine fighting over a female dog in season would cease if they had both dogs neutered. Mr. Curry interrupted by saying that he refused to have his dogs fixed. A discussion followed and it finally got down to an ultimatum from Mrs. Curry, "Either have both dogs neutered or give one away. Bob, you select which of our dogs must go!" Mr. Curry looked to me for help.

"Will neutering them guarantee that their fighting will cease?" I told him that it might but there was no way I could honestly make any kind of guarantee. Mrs. Curry said, "Lets have both dogs fixed." Mr. Curry hemmed and hawed and finally said, "I can't make a choice between the two dogs. We have had both of them for several years. Selecting one of them is like getting rid of a member of the family. Let's try the surgery and if that doesn't work, then we may have the make that unpleasant decision."

I reminded him that the surgery would not be effective this time for the male hormone was already in their dogs' bloodstream and it would take some time for it to dissipate. It would be best to evaluate the effects of surgery when your neighbor's dog came into heat the next time. Mr. Curry said, "Maybe if we paid the Parks to spay their dog, the problem might be resolved more easily." The Currys agreed to talk this idea over with their neighbors and possibly future situations could be averted. As they left, they were still discussing the options that had been presented. I never found out from that hospital what solution was implemented.

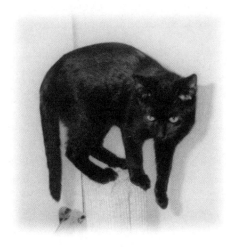

# -24-

## A SHADY SPOT

**I**t was a hot Saturday afternoon when I got my first call. I had initially started to do some yard work, but the heat of the day drove me to a lounge chair in the shade. A cool glass of iced tea was conveniently at my elbow and I was on the verge of taking a nap. A few gnats were annoying me and I swatted at them a couple of times. My eyelids were just about to close when Marna called from the door to inform me that an operator was on the line.

It was an accident case in San Pedro. I changed from my work clothes to something more suitable and sloshed some water on my face to revive me. Albert decided to join me at the last minute. We were off in a southerly direction to the harbor area.

Albert held the hospital door open, and Mr. and Mrs. Moulton brought Sparky in on a makeshift stretcher. They had covered both the plywood stretcher and Sparky with an old blanket. We took Sparky immediately into the treatment room. He made no effort to stand, but he would raise his head and attempt to look at us. Mr. Moulton looked at Sparky through tear filled eyes and said, "I feel terrible. It was all my fault."

Sparky had sought relief from the hot sun under the family car in the driveway. It was shady there and the concrete was cool. Mr. Moulton had gotten into the car and backed out over his dog. He felt the bump as the wheel passed over Sparky's body. He said, "I got out of the car and Sparky was awake but could not rise. I called to my wife to find a blanket or spread and then I got a piece of plywood and slid Sparky over on it. Then I phoned the hospital. Is he hurt badly?" "Let me see what his problem is before I made any recommendations or comments," was my response.

I examined Sparky carefully. His mucous membrane color was not bad—probably only a response to shock and not to internal hemorrhaging. His feet responded to stimulus and that lead me to think that there was no spinal damage. I started a drip of saline and dextrose and added solu-delta-cortef to counteract the effects of shock. I raised his upper rear leg and he whined and tried to raise his head again. I then put on a rubber glove and did a rectal exam. This really seemed to cause him pain.

I conferred with the Moultons and recommended an anesthetic so I could position him properly for an X ray. Albert went out to my car and brought in the gas anesthetic machine. A few minutes later Sparky was relaxed and under my control. All of us had a job. George rolled the anesthetic machine into the X-ray room, Mrs. Moulton rolled the intravenous stand, and Mr. Moulton and I carried Sparky on the stretcher. It was not as easy a task as it sounds for we had to move as a unit to insure that the intravenous and the anesthetic remained connected.

Sparky was placed on the X-ray table and the plywood and blanket were gently removed. Mr. Moulton assisted me in properly positioning Sparky so I could obtain the proper radiographic views. Several pictures were taken and twenty minutes later all of us were looking at the wet films. Sparky had a crushed pelvis and it was a bad one. Extensive surgery would be necessary. I explained the problem to the Moultons and discussed what needed to be done to return their dog to normal function—the surgical technique would be explained by their regular veterinarian. I needed to digitally expand the pelvis rectally so Sparky could defecate. The many pieces of pelvic bone would have to be aligned surgically the following morning.

The Moultons looked at each other and discussed what would be best. I just stood there waiting for their decision. Finally they asked me to step out of the room for a few minutes. When I returned they informed me that they had decided to put their male, eight-year-old mixed terrier to sleep. I nodded and stepped out of the room to prepare the necessary documents. Mr. Moulton signed them and tendered his account.

They asked if they could spend a few minutes alone with their dog. I disconnected the intravenous drip and the anesthetic machine and stepped out of the room again. About twenty minutes later they came out into the reception room and left. I connected the syringe with the euthanasia compound to the installed needle that was already taped to Sparky's leg and slowly injected the solution. Sparky gave one last breath and was relieved of his pain forever. Homeward bound, I tried to feel the remorse that the Moultons were obviously experiencing. I knew that Sparky's passing would create a void in their lives.

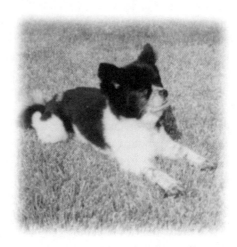

# ─────╱╲───────25─

# THE BASEBALL BAT

**T**he Eardleys were at the front desk when I entered the hospital Wednesday morning. They had brought Chum in to be neutered. Both Jo and I chatted with them and they brought us up to date regarding some of Chum's habits. "Chum likes to lay on our feet. If we are seated, he will lay on our feet and we can hardly move them. We never have cold feet anymore. Gringo used to do this, too."

"Chum loves to be outside with our boys. Whatever object they throw, whether it be a stick, ball, or block of wood, he retrieves it and drops it at the thrower's feet. He performs this task endlessly. The boys' arms tire before Chum's exuberance diminishes. One day Rob threw a stick out into an adjacent field and Chum brought back the handle of an old broken baseball bat. He would not lay it down at Rob's feet and just kept it in his mouth and looked at Rob while wagging his tail. He would not relinquish it. It was his! He had no intention of even sharing it with anyone."

Mr. Eardley had heard Rob relate the story that evening. He went over to Chum's box to investigate. The old broken bat handle had belonged to Gringo. Mr. Eardley had pitched it over the back fence when Gringo had died. Chum found it and now coveted it. When they completed the story, they reminded me that I had told them earlier that no two dogs are supposed to be alike. Chum selected the same place in the back yard as Gringo for his toilet area—under the apricot tree. The clothes pole was the place where both of them raised their leg.

As time went on, Chum would sit beside the Eardleys and rest his head on their laps when he wanted attention. He would roll his big brown eyes up at them until he attracted their attention and got his just reward for being a faithful friend—a pat on the head and maybe a scratch or two behind the ear. The Eardleys showed me a snapshot of Gringo doing the same thing. Mr. Eardley said that he would swear that Chum and Gringo were the same dog. Gringo must have come back in Chum's color pattern for that was the only difference. The size, manners, and habits all made the Eardleys think this was possible. However, none of us believed in reincarnation. We put our heads together and tried to analyze the similarity of the two pets. The shoes, bat handle, and teddy bear probably still carried a lingering scent of Gringo. The ground under the apricot tree and the clothes pole probably did also.

The other habits like fetching thrown items and placing his head on laps were performance tasks which were rewarded with kind words of encouragement or a pat on his head. We felt that Gringo had such a happy dog's life with his human family that somehow the family was able to convey to Chum these same do's and don'ts of the dog world to insure that Chum would realize as happy an existence here on earth as Gringo did. I prefer to believe that the Lord was looking down on the Eardley family and wanted them to realize that He approved of their values in life. Chum was there to share in their joy and family experiences for reasons none of us will ever understand or know.

It was almost noon when Ross stuck his head in the door to say hello. Ross was a close friend of mine from veterinary school and I had not seen him for several years. I was just filling a prescription for my last client of the morning and suggested that we go to lunch together if he could spare the time.

Ross and I had gone in different directions in our practice lives. Ross had large animal interests while I sought a career in small animal medicine. He said that he was free all afternoon and would be delighted to join me only if he could buy lunch. I argued with him but finally relinquished the honor. We agreed on a local Mexican restaurant to satisfy our hunger pangs.

We had been close comrades in school and our wives were close friends as well. We talked of our families and our progeny—he had two girls and I had three sons. He resided in the country and I in the city suburbs.

Finally our conversation settled around our escapades in veterinary school. We spent most of the time studying and had little time for social activities because we carried from eighteen to twenty-three units each semester and this kept our noses in the books. However to break the rigors of studying, we were always open to some levity. Even though hours were spent studying we tried to have a good time—many such incidents were at each other's expense. After awhile our conversation got around to some of the pranks we pulled on each other as well as some of the ones we instituted on our classmates.

"Remember the time someone put some horse manure in my tobacco pouch?" I remarked. "Yeah, I had a hard time mixing it so that you wouldn't discover it." I interrupted Ross at this stage by saying, "Now I finally have found out who the culprit was. It took you almost fifteen years to admit you were the perpetrator." Ross laughed and said, "I believed you knew all the time. I knew that you suspected me but as long as you did not know for certain, you didn't try to seek revenge."

We had started out with a margarita apiece and decided to get another when Ross suggested we get a pitcher instead. After all he had the afternoon free. I could only remember two scheduled appointments so I called Jo and asked her to reschedule them. The entire afternoon was now ours. We talked about the fall of both our junior and senior years when we leased a field by the Sacramento River when ducks were migrating. Six of us built duck blinds and that gave us three shooting spots to share during the season. Several times we also went pheasant hunting. These outings supplied us some excitement as well as relief from the rigors of studying.

Ross and I remembered the time the head of a large animal clinic came into the veterinary library and told us to do a caesarean section on a ewe. This was unheard of for junior students and reserved for the senior class but no seniors could be found and surgery needed to be done.

We talked about many things and provoked our memories to recall others. It was almost five o'clock when I decided to look at my watch. I called Jo to see how everything had gone at the hospital in my absence. She had rescheduled the two afternoon appointments and made several more for the next day. I had numerous phone calls to make on the following day as well. Marna had called and Jo told her I went out to lunch with a former classmate named Ross. Marna told Jo that I wouldn't be back very early and she was right.

Ross left for home and I got home to have dinner with Marna and the boys on time. Fortunately there were no emergencies that night so I was able to get a good night's sleep before my busy day began when the sun came up.

# —26—

# THREE-TOED CAT

**I**t had been drizzling all day and as I pulled into the driveway, it finally commenced raining hard. It had been a trying day at the office and it was great to be home. I looked forward to a relaxing evening after one of Marna's scrumptious home-cooked meals. Allen had already started a fire in the fireplace and my leather chair next to the fire looked very inviting. Greta had been in the bedroom with the boys and had come out to greet me. She then squeezed herself between my chair and the fireplace in order to soak up the warmth. I gave her a pat, settled into my chair, then kicked off my shoes and stretched.

Marna brought me a cup of her special hazelnut coffee to sip before dinner, which was only a few moments away. I had a few minutes' catnap before George informed me that dinner was ready. I took my seat at the head of the table and asked Albert to say grace as we held hands and thanked our Lord for his bountiful blessing.

Marna had just placed the roast on the table when the phone rang. I was hoping that it would not be for me and was disappointed when informed that the San Pedro answering service wished to speak to me. They briefly explained what they thought the problem was and then connected me to the Jeffersons.

Their Collie, Baron, had a very sore "thing." He was constantly licking himself at his male parts and would not allow any of the family to check him at that location. He appeared to be very swollen in that area and he was definitely uncomfortable. I realized that it was not an immediate emergency and set the time to meet them in an hour. This would give me time to enjoy supper and not have to hurry in the rain to San Pedro. I completed dinner and was on my way—so much for a quiet evening by the fire.

Mrs. Jefferson was waiting in her car out of the rain when I arrived. She brought Baron in and apologized for not having any help as her husband was out of town on business. I recorded the necessary information and entered the dog's age as six years. As he walked into the treatment room, I noticed that he was somewhat stiff in his rear legs. This was a sure sign of his discomfort, which was confirmed when he tried to stop twice and lick his prepuce.

As I bent over to pick him up, he growled at me. At the same time, Mrs. Jefferson notified me that he was not a friendly dog. With this information I stepped out of the room and found a muzzle. I asked the owner to place it over his mouth and tighten it. When this was accomplished, I lifted him up on the table and just ignored his complaining growl.

He was too big and strong for Mrs. Jefferson to hold so I suggested that it would be best to sedate him. She gave me permission and soon I was looking at a very relaxed Collie. I raised his upper leg and found a large abscess near his penis. His temperature was over 103 degrees and that helped confirm my diagnosis. I took a large needle and tapped the swollen area, and pus oozed out of the needle hub. I asked Mrs. Jefferson to wait in the reception room while I attended to the abscess.

The abscess was lanced and more than a cup of purulent matter was collected in the abscess pan. Floating in the middle of the discharge was a foxtail. I lavaged the area with sterile saline and swabbed it with a weak solution of tincture of iodine before infusing some antibiotic ointment into the lesion. I then established a seton drain to allow any more of the purulent matter to be discharged.

I invited the owner to the back of the hospital to demonstrate how Baron needed to be treated at home. The phone rang. Marna said to call the Redondo Beach exchange. I told her that I was busy and couldn't make the return call at that moment but asked her to call the operator and tell her that I would contact her in about ten minutes.

After showing Mrs. Jefferson the treatment procedure, she said, "He'll never let me do it." She wanted to know if I could keep him in the hospital for a day or two until her husband returned home. I quoted the hospitalization fee and she readily agreed to it. Besides, she informed me, it was too repulsive for her to tend to the abscess in the manner I had demonstrated.

Baron was waking up so I quickly fixed a cage for him in the treatment ward and placed him in it. I also made out a cage card and put a warning star on it to indicate that he might be dangerous to handle and to be careful. Mrs. Jefferson left the required deposit and thanked me for warning the morning staff about Baron's temperament. She said, "I'd feel terrible if he bit anyone."

I escorted my client to her car under the protection of my umbrella before turning to the task of cleaning up the mess. All of the instruments were put into a disinfectant solution and allowed to stand for the morning staff to sterilize. The treatment table was washed down and disinfected. When all was cleaned up, I called the Redondo Beach operator. She had Mrs. James on the line who had just called back to cancel her emergency because she did not wish to wait any longer but since I was now available, she rescinded her cancellation attempt and was connected to me. The James's cat had an injured toe on his front foot. I agreed to meet her at the Redondo Beach hospital in a few minutes.

I was unlocking the front door of the hospital when Mrs. James arrived. She was a client of that hospital so I located Zip's card in the files and we went into the exam room. Zip, a male tabby cat, had a toe that was about five times its normal size. He could only walk on that foot with difficulty. Zip had a high temperature to go with his swollen toe. I was looking at my second abscess of the night.

I gave Zip a sedative and took him into the treatment room to lance the swollen foot. Considerable pus was discharged. In manipulating the toe, I noted that the bone in that toe was broken. I returned to the front room where Mrs. James was waiting and explained the situation to her. An X ray was taken and several bone fragments were noted in the fracture site. I showed the radiograph to Mrs. James and recommended that the infected toe be amputated. With purulent matter in the fracture site, it was unlikely that the bone would never heal properly. She agreed.

The gas machine was brought in and Zip was entubated and connected to the anesthetic. I set out the needed instruments pack and was preparing to glove up when Mrs. James knocked on the surgery room door. She had decided to go home but wanted to first relate to me how the injury may have occurred. "Zip is a hunter. He always brings his trophies to the back door. Four days ago he was proudly sitting beside a gopher and was licking this paw. Could the gopher have bitten him hard enough to break a bone?" I responded by saying that anything is possible if the conditions are right. I escorted her to her car under my umbrella and then locked myself in and prepared for surgery.

It was necessary to make my amputation incision as far away from the infected area as possible. The bone was then cleanly severed and tissue was used to cover the end of the severed bone to provide padding. Skin was united and my surgery was completed. I was now looking at a three-toed cat. I injected an antibiotic into the muscle to discourage any infection and then made Zip a resident of the treatment ward. The hospital was cleaned up and I headed for home.

It was still raining hard and the roads were slick so I drove especially carefully. My route took me by Marie Callender's so I stopped and purchased a whole apple pie. Marna had just tucked the boys in and heard their prayers when I came into the house. I whispered to her about the pie and she decided to save it for the next night's dessert as it was too late for the boys to indulge in anything right now. We went out into the family room with a cup of coffee while we enjoyed the fire and listened to the beat of rain on the roof. I remarked to Marna that the pie on the kitchen counter certainly smelled good. She took my remark as a request, and in a few minutes she was returning with a piece of apple pie for each of us. Greta was even convinced that she deserved a bite—she stared at us while we ate, making us feel uncomfortable.

# —27—

# A RESCUE CASE

**I**t was Sunday morning again and time for my treatment rounds at four hospitals. I was up early and on my way after stopping in the kitchen long enough to fill my traveling cup with coffee before I headed for the door.

I arrived at the Hawthorne hospital, put on a smock, and checked the cases that would require my attention. When I do treatments, the closing staff on Saturday will usually leave the necessary cards on the counter with any notes attached to them for my edification. Three cards awaited me.

One cat needed an antibiotic injection and its abscess treated, a Llasso Apso needed the sutures on his shoulder checked, and the last patient, a white Persian cat, needed its eyes treated. The first two patients were quickly treated and I went into the second ward to get Snowball, the white Persian, and found the cage door ajar and the cage empty. I did not have time to hunt for her so I closed every door I could in the hospital and divided a can of cat food into six portions and put those portions into throw away food dishes. I then distributed the six portions in various places throughout the hospital that seemed likely hiding places for a frightened feline. My goal was to see which dish had been emptied and then to search that area when I returned later. I left a note for the kennel staff stating that the Morans' cat, Snowball, was loose somewhere in the hospital and to close all doors and leave the food as I had placed it on the floor.

I next went to Torrance and treated a dog with a foxtail abscess on its foot and another dog that had gastro-intestinal problems. I was soon on my way to my next stop at San Pedro where I had only one patient to see. The dog had a lesion on its back. A large collar was on the dog indicating to me that it had either been licking or scratching at the sore. I rubbed in some ointment and cleaned the cage as the note attached to the card said that no staff would be in on this Sunday. This meant that I was to feed the dog that morning and again in the evening.

I returned to the Hawthorne hospital to check on my escapee. The cleaning staff had come and gone. None of the food in the dishes that I had left had been touched. I headed for Manhattan Beach for my final scheduled treatment stop of the morning. The staff was still there and they assisted me by bringing the cases to the treatment table while the other staff workers cleaned the vacated cage and put in food and fresh water.

I was slightly ahead of my schedule of meeting Marna and the boys at church so I stopped by the Hawthorne hospital again to see if any of the food had been eaten. The dish in the pharmacy was completely empty. Snowball could not be in either the cabinets or the cupboards for their doors were still tightly closed. She had to be behind the refrigerator. I took off the front panel and could not see her. I slid the refrigerator forward and found her crouching in the corner behind it. She was covered with dust and lint. I had no intention of bathing her so I relocated her in her original cage that the staff had cleaned. I left a note indicating what had happened and suggested a courtesy bath on Monday morning. I collected all of the food dishes and combined them before putting them into Snowball's cage for her to indulge in.

I headed directly for church. Marna had taken Albert to his Sunday School class and sent the older two to theirs. I quickly located Marna in the area where we frequently sit and joined her in the first hymn of the morning. After church we gathered up the boys and headed for home. We broke tradition by not eating Sunday brunch at a restaurant and instead headed home for Marna had planned a special breakfast.

The boys had finished eating and were now occupied playing a board game. Marna and I were enjoying another cup of coffee and just relaxing when Bob Truffit called me direct. He was calling from a private residence along the Palos Verdes Peninsula.

Bob's dog, Pete, had just fallen about thirty feet down a cliff and the fire department had been called to rescue him. As soon as Pete was topside again, Bob wanted me to examine him for any possible injuries. At this moment, Pete was lying motionless on a ledge about halfway down the cliff to the ocean below.

I left right away for the Palos Verdes hospital where Bob was a client. He was a close church friend and knew my home number. He thought it would save time by circumventing the emergency operator.

I got to the hospital and had ample time to get a cage prepared for my incoming patient. Bob and Pete arrived about forty minutes later. Pete was wrapped up in a blanket provided by the fire department and secured with straps on plywood stretcher. Pete was motionless except for his eyes and his expanding chest when he breathed. His eyes followed me as I walked around the treatment table.

I started an intravenous drip and added medication to it to counteract shock. When the syringe and tubing were secured to Pete's front leg, it was time to determine if there were any fractures. Bob helped me position Pete on the X-ray table and I took several views of Pete's chest, abdomen, and appendages. As each film was developed, Bob and I would scan it to determine what damage had occurred. After scrutinizing six radiographs, I could not find any evidence of a fracture. Some density was noted in both the chest and abdominal areas and that was more than likely related to the impact of the fall when Pete's internal organs were slammed against his body wall.

The drip was adjusted to six drops per minute. Bob rolled the intravenous stand into the intensive care ward and I carried the Weimaraner and placed him on the towels that I had previously prepared for him. Bob and I then left Pete in his cage and retired to the reception desk where I needed to record some information. Pete was a five-year-old male and had been well trained as a hunting dog. Bob had taken Pete for a walk along the cliff area and when they got to a remote area, Bob released Pete from the leash so he could roam about and get some exercise. Pete had flushed some doves and had raced after them unaware of the edge of the cliff. Soon he was airborne.

"I raced over expecting to see Pete on the rocks a hundred or so feet below, but there he was on a ledge just below the crest. There was no way I could get to him so I walked over to the nearest house and borrowed their phone to first call the fire department and then you.

"The fire department responded right away and one of the men rappelled down and lifted Pete onto a basket that had been lowered. It was lucky that he had been knocked out by the fall or he might have moved and fallen the rest of the way to the ocean below. Quite a group of people had gathered to watch the recovery event. I don't know who supplied the stretcher but the recovery team furnished the blanket and straps.

"Several people assisted in carrying Pete to the road where my car was located. I was glad to have all of that help since Pete weighs over seventy pounds. I thanked the firemen and those around me who assisted and was on my way to meet you."

We returned to intensive care and checked on Pete. I suggested to Bob that he might as well go home. I planned to stay and keep an eye on his dog for awhile. Bob suggested we stroll down to the corner for a sandwich and coffee break. Before we left he felt it prudent to call home and tell Joyce about Pete and his problem.

When we returned to the hospital, Pete's vital signs had improved immensely; they were almost in the normal range. I connected another liter of fluid to the drip setup and again added a vial of solu-delta-cortef to continue our struggle against the shock syndrome. Pete raised his head and looked at Bob when he heard Bob mention his name. Bob was greatly relieved. I told Bob that I would check on Pete later and would phone him and give him an up to the minute report.

I had two more emergencies that afternoon and night before I got back to the hospital to check on Pete. Pete was no longer on his side but was resting on his chest. He raised his head when I opened the ward door. I checked his vital signs again. His mucous membranes now were a nice pink color. This indicated to me that the possibility of any serious internal bleeding was minimal. I called the Truffit's home and they were delighted with the progress report.

On my way to my hospital Monday morning, I stopped by to see Pete again. He was standing. His stance indicated that he was very stiff and sore. I called Bob and brought him up to date. Bob said, "I don't think the fall hurt him one bit. The sudden stop did all of the damage." We could jest about the accident now that the outcome was favorable. I explained to Bob that the attending doctor would go over the radiographs with a fine toothed comb to see if anything detrimental had occurred because a dry film is much easier to read. I asked him to call the hospital about ten that morning and talk to the attending veterinarian.

# —∧— 28—

# A PLAYGROUND SLIDE

The boys, Allen, George, and Albert, were playing catch in the cul-de-sac where we lived. Albert, the youngest, was not as proficient as his brothers but was delighted to be a participant. Actually he was the go-getter. Whoever missed a catch would ask Albert to retrieve it. He soon tired of this and went and got Greta, our German Shorthair Pointer, who was excited to join in the activities. All went well until Allen noticed that prominent teeth marks were on the surface of the leather hard ball. He instructed Albert to pen Greta up again. Albert refused.

Soon three boys and a dog were walking through the gate. A squabble had ensued and I left the Saturday football game I was watching on television to help them resolve their disagreement. As I got up from my chair, the phone rang. I was connected to Mr. Conyer whose dog had been injured in an accident and needed medical attention. I asked George to go with me and that appeared to stop the argument for he was the most vociferous of the three. Soon the two of us were on our way to Manhattan Beach.

I unlocked the front door and George turned on the lights. Momentarily the Conyers appeared with Taco, a Chihuahua. The left front leg was obviously broken and Taco was in considerable pain. I sedated Taco to relieve his discomfort and then proceeded with the necessary X rays. Both the radius and ulna were fractured at midshaft. No bone fragments were evident and I explained that it was a relative easy fracture to repair.

120

I thought about placing a splint on the foreleg and having the resident veterinarian do the surgery Sunday morning when he came in for treatments. I opened the appointment book to schedule surgery and noticed my name. I then remembered that it was a three day weekend and I was taking both Sunday and Monday morning treatments. It was too long to wait for Tuesday surgery. I explained this to the Conyers and they wanted me to do the surgery either Sunday or Monday morning if it was possible. I felt that it would be best to take Taco right into surgery since he was already sedated.

George brought in the anesthetic machine and we connected Taco while we could do so without any further sedation. I spent a few moments with the Conyers explaining my proposed technique and let them know I would call them after surgery. George locked the front door after the Conyers left and then called his mother to tell her that I would be in surgery for awhile.

While the surgery room was properly set up for orthopedic repair, George had trimmed Taco's fur from the proposed surgical site. I scrubbed the surgical area and moved the anesthetic machine and Taco from treatment to surgery. George brought in the radiographs and placed them on the view screen for my perusal during surgery.

An incision was made at the appropriate location and the fractured ends of the bones were exposed. A steel pin was inserted into the center of the ulna and the bone was pinned using the retrograde procedure. Now the ulna was in proper position. The ulna now acted as a spacer for the radius enabling the radius to align in correct position. The tip of the exposed pin was cut off about one and a half inches from the skin surface so it could be recovered when the bone had healed sufficiently. Next the suture site was closed. The leg was splinted with a walking splint and padded and taped to the splint in such a manner that the leg could not rotate. George had already prepared a cage with several layers of towels and put a pan of water in for Taco. I disconnected the Chihuahua from the gas machine and George took him into the recovery ward and placed him in the assigned cage.

George commenced the cleanup and I called the Conyers to give them a report on Taco's surgery. I finally had time to find out how the accident occurred. Mrs. Conyers explained that the family had gone to a local park for a picnic and some activity for the children. Taco went along on a leash to be with the family members. The children enjoyed the jungle gym. "The children were racing to see who could make the most trips down the slide. They came up with the idea of taking their large ball down the slide with them and rolling over it at the bottom of the slide. Like all children, this novelty soon wore off. They looked around for something new to do that was exciting. They asked if they could take Taco down the slide with them. We saw no harm if they promised to hold him securely on their laps. Taco did not like the first ride at all. On his second forced journey, he jumped off our son's lap and slid down the slide by himself ahead of Tommy. Tommy then landed on Taco. Taco yelped and came over to us. I know we should have used better judgement, but that is in retrospect."

By the time I got off the phone, George had the surgery area as clean as when we first used it. The surgery pack was ready for sterilization and I put it into the autoclave. George called his mother to let her know we were out of surgery and then we walked down to the fast-food restaurant on the corner to indulge in a soft drink.

When we got back to the hospital, the autoclave needed venting. I asked George to call home and check with his mother. I had two calls pending. One was at Torrance and the second at Hawthorne. I called the specific answering services and obtained the clients' telephone numbers and then called them to set up a time to meet them at the respective hospitals. The Hawthorne case was scheduled first as it was nearby and only fifteen minutes away. We arrived first and waited a few minutes before the Clevengers pulled into the parking lot and brought in the most bedraggled Cocker that I had ever seen. The patient record was filled out. I was introduced to Frisco officially. He was a blond four-year-old male.

Their complaint was that Frisco was chewing her feet and shaking her head. Besides all of that, she had a very offensive body odor. The odor was evident to both George and me and even caused George to curl up his nose as we went into the exam room. I nodded to George to pick up Frisco and put him on the exam table. He was not happy with my request but did as I had asked. He held Frisco securely as I proceeded with my examination.

Three of Frisco's feet showed evidence of foxtail abscesses. His ears were so painful that he objected violently whenever they were touched. I put that portion of the examination on hold, too. His skin was still another problem. Several large hair mats covered his body—on his rump, left shoulder, and on his chest. I got the clippers out and was able to trim the hair enough to see what lay under these tight hair mats. Foxtails were everywhere. These weed seeds had penetrated the skin in numerous places and caused fetid smelling sores. I showed these lesions to the Clevengers and they looked at each other and said nothing. I berated them for allowing Frisco to get into such a condition.

"This is your dog, isn't it?" I asked.

They responded in the affirmative.

"You noticed that I did not say pet, didn't you?"

They then gave another affirmative response and then asked, "Why?"

"Pets are not treated the way Frisco has been. They are part of the family and are treated accordingly."

The Clevengers remained quiet.

I continued by saying that they should be ashamed of Frisco's condition. "Frisco needs considerable care right now!"

"What do you recommend?" asked Mr. Clevenger.

"I need to anesthetize Frisco. Then I will check his feet for foxtails, trim the mats of hair, and treat the sores underneath. His ears need to be cleaned and packed as well. In fact, it would be best to give Frisco a close trim all over followed with a medicated bath."

"Please go ahead and do what you recommended. When will he be able to go home?"

"Let's see, this is a Saturday of a three-day holiday weekend. I could discharge her tomorrow morning when I come in to do treatments. I will call and tell you when I arrive at the hospital and then if you would come down right away for her, I would appreciate it because I have several hospitals to do treatments early that morning."

The Clevengers agreed with that arrangement and left the hospital. I called the Torrance exchange and asked them to call the next client and extend the appointment about an hour.

George and I went to work. He held Frisco and I sedated him and passed an endotracheal tube. Then George went to my car and brought in the gas machine and we connected Frisco to it. It took some time to clip Frisco. George manned the vacuum. Soon all of the mats had been trimmed as well as his ears and feet. I started with the ears first. Several foxtails were found in each ear and the ears were infected. The ears were treated and then the antibiotic, panalog, was infused into each ear. Two of his feet had to be lanced to remove the foxtails. Setons were applied there. His third foot had foxtails but they had not penetrated too deeply and I was able to grasp them with forceps and remove them. I disconnected the anesthetic so Frisco could begin waking up.

His skin was a major problem. Under the mats, the skin was a mess. Foxtails had penetrated through the mats and they looked like a forest of trees. We removed them carefully and treated the sores with antibiotics. Several other smaller mats were discovered and they were treated in the same manner. A foxtail was even discovered and removed from his right eye. When we were satisfied that all of these foreign bodies had been removed and treated, we put Frisco into the tub and George commenced giving him a much needed medicated bath.

While he was soaking in a lathered condition in the tub, I made the entries on the patient card and George prepared a cage in the treatment room. After the bath, the lesions were again treated and Frisco received both a cortisone and an antibiotic injection. George toweled him down and placed him in the cage and we were on our way to Torrance.

At Torrance, Mr. Sheffield had already arrived. I apologized for the delay. The client seemed to understand. Bogey, a boxer, had a cut on his hip that needed suturing. Bogey was a very active dog and I did not feel that I would be able to apply sutures with only a local anesthetic block. George again assisted me while I administered surital. The hip was clipped and scrubbed. I then debrided the lesion and applied eight to ten stainless steel sutures to the gaping wound because the owner said that Bogey had chewed out his stitches on a previous occasion. At this stage, Bogey was raising his head and trying to look around at us. I told Mr. Sheffield that Bogey could stay here overnight and be discharged on Sunday or he could go home if Mr. Sheffield felt he could handle the dog. Mr. Sheffield opted to take his dog home. George held Bogey on the table while Mr. Sheffield took care of his account and then I carried the waking dog out to the car. George and I returned the hospital to normal and soon we were heading for home.

It was now dark and the moon was illuminating the south bay. We thought of stopping for a bite to eat but rationalized that Marna would see to it that some supper had been set aside for our indulgence.

Sunday morning I was up early doing treatments at various hospitals. Just before I left San Pedro, I called the Clevengers and told them I would be at the Hawthorne hospital in fifteen minutes. They were waiting for me when

I arrived. Frisco was discharged after I had written several prescriptions and given them instructions for their use. I apologized for being so adamant about the care Frisco needed. (I had been on the verge of rudeness). I politely explained that Frisco did need more attention than he had been receiving and that he should be close-clipped about every six months to avoid repetition of this foxtail problem. They paid their bill, thanked me, and left. I never expected to see the Clevengers again and I now felt badly about the tone of my voice when Frisco had first been admitted.

I got home about nine-thirty and changed before heading for church. We usually sit in a certain area and I located Marna quickly. I had to sit behind her and she did not know I was present for a few minutes until we were asked to introduce ourselves to those seated near us. After church, I treated the family to brunch at a local restaurant. I checked with the four answering services so they would be able to contact me in an emergency. We had a great meal and I was not called by any of the operators while there.

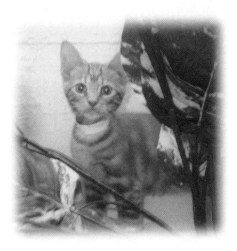

# —⋀——29–

# A Vicious Pit Bull

I had responded to an emergency at the Hawthorne hospital. On the exam table in front of me was a large gray, altered, male cat named Avis. Avis had a broken left front leg. The fracture was in the vicinity of his elbow. Mr. and Mrs. Davis had brought their cat in after it had hopped through its cat door and then limped across the kitchen floor on three legs as it headed for his cat basket in the corner of the room. Mrs. Davis had wrapped Avis in a blanket, and I carefully exposed his leg. I confirmed that their tentative diagnosis was correct when I palpated it and felt crepitation [bones rubbing together].

We went into the X-ray room and took anterior, posterior, lateral, and oblique views. We looked at the radiographs on the view screen and found that Avis had an olecranon [elbow] fracture of a serious nature. Both of the lateral condyles [articular part of the joint] of the humerus were separated. This meant that they would have to be held tightly together with a condylar clamp while a bone screw was used to keep them in that position as the bones healed.

Mrs. Davis and her husband consulted and she said, "Go ahead and put A. D. back together again." I looked up and said, "You just told me your cat's name was Avis." Mr. Davis smiled and said, "We call him Avis Davis and shorten it to A. D. on occasion."

I informed them that it would be a long surgery, so Mrs. Davis restrained Avis on the exam table while her husband gave me necessary information for the patient card and left a deposit. Before they left I connected Avis to the anesthetic machine, then took him into treatment room for surgical prep. Avis's leg was clipped, scrubbed, and swabbed with an antiseptic solution. Surgery was started. The condyles were aligned and the condylar clamp held them tightly in the proper position. A trans-condylar screw was affixed to hold the fragments of bone in place. When the clamp was removed there was a slight rotation of the fragments so positioning pins were placed on each side to hold the fracture in the correct alignment for healing.

A post X ray was taken to confirm the proper fixation and then a supportive splint was positioned on the leg to insure that the elbow would not move. Any movement might cause the weaker fragments of bone to crack or splinter. If this happened, Avis could limp for the rest of his cat years.

Avis was put into a recovery cage and I spent a half hour making up the surgery pack and putting it into the autoclave. Surgery was cleaned and all of the splint material was put in its proper drawer. I took the anesthetic machine out to the car and returned to the hospital. I noted that A. D. was waking up and trying to figure out what had happened. His leg with the splint was about an inch longer than his good leg and he was having a diffi-cult time trying to get up into a sitting position with the awkward apparatus attached to his leg. Finally he made it and then glanced at me with a bewildered look.

I called the Davis household and informed them that Avis had come through surgery in a fine manner. I informed them that if the leg healed properly, A. D. would probably not limp at all—only time would tell. It would be very important for them to keep Avis as quiet as possible in order for proper healing to take place. They thanked me again. I asked them to call in the morning and the resident doctor would fill them in with the details about their cat's aftercare.

I had a call from the Gardena hospital service and a Mr. Queensley wanted to talk to me. He had not given the operator any clues as to his problem but he seemed quite irritated when I was connected. The first thing he said was, "Doc, I want you to put my dog down!"

"Is he injured?" I asked.

"No, he is just ill tempered. He wants to fight and kill anything that has four feet. He is difficult to coop-up and extremely hard to restrain. It is impossible to separate him from another dog because he is so aggressive."

"How is he around people?"

"That is what worries me. He almost turned on me tonight. He killed the neighbor's dog about an hour ago and then made a pass at me when I tried to pull him off."

"I am sorry to hear that," I remarked.

"Both a police officer and a humane officer were at my house this evening and advised me to have this done. The owner of the dog he killed had his dog on a leash on the sidewalk when Bozo broke out of the backyard and killed him. My Pit Bull is just too dangerous to own. I will have a lawsuit on my hands before the week is out. I am afraid he might attack a child if he gets too excited."

I agreed to meet them at the Gardena hospital in forty minutes. Bozo was waiting at the door with Mr. Queensley when I pulled into the driveway. Bozo growled at me and I gave him a wide birth and unlocked the hospital. Bozo was not afraid of me. I kept one eye on him for my own safety—after all, I had been warned.

I asked Mr. Queensley to put Bozo up on the treatment table but he could not lift his eighty-plus pounds dog by himself. Bozo continually faced me when I attempted to circle him to lift up his back end. He knew something was up and now was growling and showing his teeth at me now whenever I moved. I backed off.

"Would Bozo eat some dog food?" I asked.

"Yes, he will probably wolf it down."

I returned with a pan of canned dog food that had been laced with ample tranquilizer tablets of acepromazine to make him sleepy. I handed the pan to the client and left the room. In a minute I was informed that the pan was empty so I had Mr. Queensley lead Bozo into the treatment ward with the intention of putting him into a lower level cage while the medication took effect. That was a mistake. A cat and two dogs occupied some of the cages and when Bozo smelled them and then saw them, he went crazy. He went out of his mind and broke loose from his owner and tried to tear the metal doors off of the cages to get at the hospitalized pets. Both of us tried to pull Bozo off but our efforts were in vane. We actually feared for our own safety. Finally Bozo quieted down and sat there and just looked at his frightened opponents. Next he lay down and watched them. The tranquilizer was beginning to take effect.

Ten minutes later I slipped a muzzle over Bozo's mouth and together we lifted the large dog up on the treatment table. I questioned Mr. Queensley about Bozo. "Has he bitten anyone?"

"No, not that I know of."

I injected the euthanasia solution into Bozo's blood stream. I told Mr. Queensley that I should hold Bozo for three to four days until I was certain that no one had been bitten. He said, "Fine." Since he had completed the paperwork and paid for my services, he left for home. I felt that he had a relieved look on his face as he exited the hospital.

I put Bozo in a cadaver bag and put him in a lower cage. I left a note asking the staff veterinarian to call me first thing in the morning. I also left a note on Bozo's bag stating, "Do not dispose of this dog." When the doctor called me the next morning, I suggested that he call the County Health Department and explain the situation that I had related to him. I said that it would be best to follow any advice the county recommended.

I got home and was still a bit shaky from my experience. I guess that Marna noticed it when she first saw me and asked, "What happened! Are you alright?" I told her the story of my evening's experience with Bozo. Marna comforted me by saying, "The community is relieved of a potentially vicious dog. You performed a necessary service."

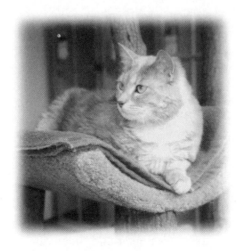

# —30—

# GRANDCHILD CONFUSION

**I** was telling Jo about the events of my previous night when Mr. Beech entered the hospital. He was carrying a cage with a hamster inside of it. He felt that it was an emergency and wanted me to take a peek at Dog. Mr. Beech was a retired fireman and about eighty years in age. He frequently walked past my hospital and would stop in for a visit if no clients were in the reception room. He always had a new story to relate to us about pets or veterinarians.

Today he had a problem with his hamster. Dog, the hamster, had a large swelling on his underside that had been abraded. It was bleeding and attracted Mr. Beech's attention. The growth had been there for some time and I had seen it before. Now Dog had scraped it and it needed attention. Jo brought Dog into the treatment room and held the hamster while I cauterized the lesion electrically. I then bandaged the hamster so that the lesion would be protected. Dog was returned to his cage and taken out to the reception room to Mr. Beech.

Jo said, "That's a strange name to call a hamster." Mr. Beech said, "I also have a rabbit named Cat, a dog named Rabbit, and a cat called Hamster." Both Jo and I shook our heads in disbelief.

"You know," he said, "When my grandchildren come over, I have a lot of fun confusing them with the names of the pets in my menagerie. When I ask one of the kids to go get Rabbit and they bring me the rabbit, I kid them and say that's Cat—that's not Rabbit. When I ask them to bring me

Dog, and they bring me the hamster, I kid them and tell them that they don't know the difference between a dog and a hamster. This game can go on for a long period of time. By the time their visit is over, they are completely confused. It takes my daughter several days to correct the problem I created with her children." Jo and I both laughed at his story. Mr. Beech continued, "I was put in place by my oldest grandchild when I asked her to bring me Dog. She put her hands on her hips and said 'Grandpa, do you want the real dog or the one you call Dog?'"

It was a good time to have a little levity at the beginning of the day. Jo said, "I think I am as confused as his grandchildren."

It was several months after I had embarrassed the Clevengers about the care of their Cocker, Frisco, when they walked in the door. They had tried to locate me because they wanted to show me how they had improved their care of Frisco. Frisco followed them in on a leash. Frisco could have been a candidate for a dog show. He strutted and held his head high. He was proud of his appearance as so were the Clevengers. Mrs. Clevenger thanked me for being so candid about my feelings concerning Frisco's previous condition. They said that I wasn't really rude but just factual. They didn't like hearing what I told them but they realized that someone had to address them in a forceful manner. They were so proud of what they had accomplished that they spent time locating me to just show off their efforts.

I arrived home that evening to be greeted by the sound of the telephone as I entered the house. The operator had a client on the line whose dog had just been bitten by a rattlesnake. I was connected to Mr. Justin without further delay.

"This is the doctor speaking."

"Hi, this is Eric Justin. My dog, Jupiter, has just been bitten by a rattlesnake."

"Are you certain that it was a rattlesnake?"

"Absolutely. I killed it and have it in a box."

"I will meet you at the San Pedro hospital right away. I will have to locate an antivenom kit before I leave."

I called the Harbor-UCLA Medical Hospital in Carson. They had kits available and I asked to have one ready as I would be there in about ten minutes. I picked up the kit and paid them the ninety dollars and was on my way to San Pedro. I arrived there thirty minutes after I had left home. The Justins were waiting.

Jupiter's shoulder was already beginning to swell and the venom was turning the tissue around the bite wound black. I infused the area with antivenom as well as some steroid and then kenneled Jupiter for awhile. They informed me that their dog was bitten in their own backyard.

"Doctor, why did you have to go by the UCLA Medical center to pick up the medication?"

"Antivenom is very expensive and it is a short-dated product. Most veterinary clinics can't afford to stock it routinely because it might expire before it is needed."

"How much does it cost?"

I showed him the receipt and explained that the kit cost the same for animals as for humans. He was very surprised.

I thought that it would be best for them to leave Jupiter for awhile. I would talk to the owners later. I kept Jupiter under observation for a period of time and when the swelling appeared to have stopped progressing, I too left for home. Later that night, I asked Allen to accompany me back to San Pedro to check on my patient. I infused more steroid around the bite wounds while Allen held him securely. I then called the Justins to give them a follow-up report.

I suggested that Jupiter could go home now if they watched him carefully and called me if they had any questions. They said that they were just leaving for a party and would not be able to keep their dog under observation.

"Would it be alright to keep Jupiter there overnight?"

"Yes. I will check him again before the office opens in the morning."

"Thanks. I will call in the morning and talk to our doctor."

"Good. He will bring you up to date and give you his input. He will tell you when he plans to discharge your pet."

Allen and I stopped at the local pizza parlor and took a pizza home for all of the family to enjoy. Allen carried it into the house and immediately attracted a lot of attention from his brothers. Marna opened a large bottle of diet soda and we carried our pizza out to the patio where it was cooler. Greta spent her time watching us enjoy our snack. We completed our treat and offered Greta some of the crust which she devoured without chewing it one bit. George thought that Greta had been slighted so he went inside and brought out some dog biscuits, which pleased Greta immensely.

# 31—

## A HEART PROBLEM

**M**rs. Dryfus was on the line. They owned a Keeshond that had collapsed while chasing a cat out of their backyard. Initially they had thought that Fritz had dropped dead, but when they carried him into the house, they realized he had a heartbeat and very shallow breathing. It was dusk on Friday night and they wanted to meet me at the Manhattan Beach hospital. I told them that I was twenty-five minutes away and if the traffic was heavy, maybe a few minutes more.

The Dryfuses were standing at the front door ringing the bell when I arrived. Mr. Dryfus held Fritz in his arms. We went into the treatment room. Fritz had a normal temperature. Auscultation [listening to sounds] of the chest was perplexing to me. The sound that I was hearing with the stethoscope indicated a probable cardiovascular problem.

I began questioning the owners in the attempt to get a better history of this two-year- old dog. I asked Mr. Dryfus to explain exactly what had happened. He said, "Fritz saw a cat in the flowerbed through the sliding glass door. Fritz wanted to get out and we obliged by opening the back door. After all, we do not like the decorations that the neighborhood cats leave in our flower garden. Well, Fritz bolted out the door and made a beeline for the cat. The cat heard him coming and headed around the house and, I guess, escaped over the side fence. I left the back door ajar so that Fritz could come back in after he had chased the intruder away. Ten to fifteen minutes later he never came back into the house. I whistled

133

for him as I usually do and received no response. I went out after Mildred suggested it would be a good idea and found Fritz lying in the petunia bed on his side. His tongue was out of his mouth and gray in color and I thought he had died. I picked him up and took him into the house. It was then I realized he was still alive and called you."

I checked Fritz's tongue and it was not the nice pink color I would have preferred it to be. "Is this the first time Fritz has acted this way?" I asked.

"No. Ever since we got him as a puppy, he has acted a bit strange when he over exercises. Both Mildred and I work so Fritz is not monitored during the day. He doesn't always pass out—that has only happened twice before. Sometimes he just stands in one location like he is trying to catch his breath. When he is rested, he goes on his merry way again."

"When was the last time he had this type of problem?"

"About three weeks ago, but Mildred and I are only home at night and on the weekends."

"I would like your permission to take an X ray of Fritz's chest."

"That is fine with me," said Mrs. Dryfus.

I was leery about giving either a sedative or an anesthetic so I asked Mr. Dryfus to put on a leaded apron and gloves and help hold his dog in the proper position. When Fritz took a deep inspiration, I asked Mr. Dryfus to hold the nares [nostrils] closed so I could get an inflated radiograph of Fritz's chest. I found it necessary to take several views in order to get two satisfactory films.

I studied the wet radiographs but was not knowledgeable enough in cardiology to perceive anything drastically wrong. I decided to wait a few minutes and see about a dry film interpretation. In the meantime, I pulled several old radiographs from the files for comparison. It appeared that the right ventrical was larger than normal in proportion to the size of the heart. I confirmed this by comparing the film with those I had pulled from the old files.

The Dryfuses had retired to the reception room with Fritz while I was developing the film. I went out, pulled up a chair, and joined them. Fritz was standing now but he was not moving around to any great degree.

I said, "I think your dog may have a congenital heart problem. On the film his heart seems to me to out of proportion to a normal heart. Fritz's right ventrical is larger than it should be."

"What should we do?" asked Mrs. Dryfus.

"I think Fritz is over his current crisis. I want him to remain calm. I would like to keep him overnight at this hospital—maybe even for a couple of days. The doctor in the morning will follow up on the case and do a thorough workup. He may want to take more X rays and some other tests."

"What do you think the problem is?" said Mr. Dryfus.

"I am not certain, but it could be what is called 'tetralogy of fallot' which is a septal defect of the heart allowing both the venous and arterial blood in the heart to mix. When this happens, not enough oxygenated blood reaches the vital tissues and a pet can pass out from hypo-oxygenation."

"Is Fritz going to die?"

"I have only given you a provisional diagnosis. The doctor tomorrow morning will take over the case and be more definitive in his report to you."

Mrs. Dryfus nodded to her husband and he agreed. They asked if they could accompany their dog to where he would be kenneled and say goodnight to him. They followed me back to the treatment ward and patted Fritz while I prepared his cage, filled his water pan, and placed some food in a dish. Fritz was patted again and I placed him in the cage. (It was later confirmed that my provisional diagnosis was correct. To the best of my knowledge, Fritz was exposed to limited exercise and lived for several years).

It was past my normal bedtime but Marna and I were still up when the Torrance hospital exchange called. Mrs. Krug had a Dachshund that had a respiratory problem. Mrs. Krug had been crying and I could hear a man's voice in the background prompting her on what to say. "Please, please, see Frau tonight," she pleaded. I agreed to meet her at the Torrance hospital whose exchange had forwarded her call. They bought in Frau, a black and tan female about four years old. I could hear Frau breathing as she came through the front door. The noise she made was very profound.

"How long has she been breathing like this?" I asked as I listened to her chest with my stethoscope. "About two days and it is getting worse. We had our house tented for termites and left Frau next door with our neighbors while we stayed at a hotel. Somehow she got away from them and apparently burrowed under the canvas and was exposed to all that gas they use. We found her at the back steps when the tenting was removed two days ago. Doctor, her condition is gradually getting worse. Is there anything you can do to help her?" I said that I would like to take an X ray and evaluate my findings before I could render an opinion.

I was able to take a dorsal-ventral and a lateral view with some help from Mr. Krug. We looked at the film together. Both of Frau's lungs were very dense. It was very likely that the gas used on termites had irritated the lungs causing fluid to be exuded into the alveolar air spaces. Frau was essentially drowning.

We had put Frau into a cage while I was developing the film. We went into the ward to check on her to see if she was comfortable. Frau had died. The excitement of being at the hospital and being held for the radiographs had been too much stress for her. Her system had required more oxygen than she was able to provide from her damaged lungs. Mr. Krug put his arm around his wife and they slowly walked to the front of the hospital. Mrs. Krug broke the silence by saying, "Frau didn't suffer long. If I had known then what I know now, I would have boarded her at a kennel."

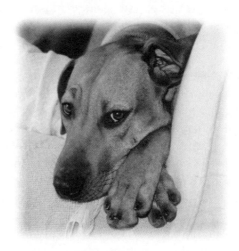

# — 32 —

# TACO BELL'S PROBLEM

**M**arna had just announced that supper was ready when the phone rang. The San Pedro exchange was on the line and they connected me to Mr. Carter. It sounded as if it was a bad case. The Carter's dog had a severe injury to one of its rear legs and Mr. Carter remarked that he hoped that I would be able to save the leg.

Marna fixed me a quick sandwich from the roast she was about to serve and then plunked it into an all too frequent sack dinner bag and handed it to me as I headed for the door. I munched my sandwich on the way to San Pedro and tried to anticipate the problem that I would have to address when I saw my evening's patient.

Mr. Carter was waiting at the hospital door with his large black Labrador, Angus, as I pulled into the parking lot. Angus's left rear leg was wrapped in a towel that was saturated with blood. We went directly into the treatment room. Information could be recorded later. Right now, Angus needed my attention. I carefully removed the towel from Angus's leg to better evaluate the injury. Blood was spurting from the wound and considerable skin was missing above the hock and the achilles tendon appeared to have been severed. Mr. Carter held Angus while I administered surital and passed the endotracheal tube. I hurried out to my car and brought in the anesthetic machine and connected Angus. Soon the Labrador was completely relaxed and my examination continued.

137

Mr. Carter appeared a little pale so I suggested he go out into the reception room and take a seat. He said that he would write his telephone number on a pad at the front desk and then go to be with his family.

I carefully searched through the tangled mass of bloody tissue and hair and either tied off the bleeding vessels or cauterized them. I debrided the ragged edges of tissue and removed all of the hair that was in the lesion. Next I searched the leg carefully to see if I could locate an artery or two that had not been damaged. One major vessel was still intact as well as several minor ones. This encouraged me that the leg might have a chance of being saved and not have to be amputated.

The tendon was sutured with stainless steel wire. Several tears had occurred in the muscle and the edges were opposed and sutured. Considerable skin tissue had to be trimmed away and this left a rather raw area at the surgical site. Furacin ointment was first applied to the exposed area and then ample gauze sponges were used to pack and protect the hock. My next task was to construct a cast so that Angus could neither flex nor extend his leg. It took me almost another hour to fit it and then adjust it to cradle the leg in the position that I desired. When all was done, I looked at Angus and was reasonable satisfied with my effort. Just as I was about to unhook the anesthetic machine, I decided that I should have a window somewhere in the distal portion of the cast to be able to ascertain if the leg remained viable. Half way down I made an opening in the cast and then I made another one more at the base of the cast where the tarsal pad was located. Now I had two windows to observe the healing progress of Angus's leg.

I disconnected Angus from the gas, administered an antibiotic, and then prepared a large padded cage for him. It took a bit of effort for me to carry the eight-five pound dog into the recovery ward and place him gently in his cage. I put the instruments into a pan to soak and made a pot of coffee before phoning the Carter house. It was a few minutes shy of midnight when I placed the call and Mr. Carter answered immediately.

I described what I had done surgically and gave the prognosis as guarded meaning that there was a chance the leg might be saved, but only a slim chance. Mr. Carter wanted to see Angus and I told him to come right down for I still had to clean up the premises and it would probably take another hour for me to do so. Fifteen minutes later, a knock on the door indicated that he had arrived.

I obtained the vital information and entered it on the patient card—black male Labrador about eight years of age. His weight was 103 pounds—I had certainly proved to be a poor judge of weight. Angus's injury was unusual. Angus would jump the six-foot block fence and visit the neighbor's rabbit hutches next door. His presence would terrify the does (females) and they would rush into their kindling box and occasionally smother their young. To correct this problem of the fence-jumping Lab, three strands of smooth wire were affixed to the top of the fence about eight inches apart. Angus tried to jump the fence again but got his rear leg tangled in the wire and hung there upside down until he was discovered. "He might have been there upside down for two or three hours," was Mr. Carter's comment. The wire had, over a period of time, sawed through the soft tissue of the leg until it reached the bone.

Keith, the resident veterinarian, would take over the case when he reported for duty later that day. It was almost two in the morning before I had put the anesthetic machine back into my car and headed for home. Keith called me later that morning and I filled him in on what I had done and told the client. He thanked me for thinking of the view windows in the cast.

Two weeks later at a local veterinary meeting, we again had an opportunity to discuss that case. The leg was still viable but healing very slowly due to the diminished blood supply. Keith had to replace the cast on two occasions because it was necessary to change the dressing around the raw areas of the hock. Each time he did this it was necessary to sedate Angus to keep him immobile.

I phoned Keith off and on for the next month or two. Finally the cast was removed and replaced with a walking splint designed for the leg. Nasty looking scars were present at the hock. Finally even the walking splint was removed. Angus exhibited a very severe limp and probably would have one for the rest of his life. He could no longer jump fences but, thank goodness, he was able to walk with all four of his feet touching the ground.

I had gotten a few hours sleep before work that morning and then an hour nap at noontime. When I stumbled through the door at home that evening I told Marna that my body needed sleep more than it needed nutrition and that I was going into the family room to take another nap. I had barely closed my eyes when the phone rang. It was six o'clock in the evening when I was alerted.

The answering service from Torrance had a Mrs. Paulos on the line about her Chihuahua that had injured itself. The operator connected me to the stressed client who informed me that her pet had either dislocated or broken its right front leg. Mrs. Paulos requested that I see her dog right away as it was in considerable pain.

I lived much closer to the hospital than the incoming client and arrived there first. I prepared to take X rays as that appeared to be necessary from our earlier telephone conversation. I pulled the Paulos's card and noted that they owned three of the breed so I was unable to complete the X-ray identification card until I knew which of her pets had sustained the injury.

Both Mr. and Mrs. Paulos arrived and introduced me to T. B. T. B. was carrying his right fore leg and refused to place it down on the exam table. I completed the X-ray card and we went into the treatment room. A mild sedative was given to relax T. B. sufficiently so we could position him properly for the X ray. Mr. Paulos held his dog in the proper way to enable me to take two views of the leg. We looked at the radiograph together. There was an obvious fracture of both the radius and ulna at the distal epiphysis. I asked if he had broken his leg before as I noticed some extra bone growth on the leg. The Paulos's said that T. B. had broken the same leg in the same place three years earlier.

I excused myself to check on the doctor's surgery schedule for the following morning. My name was on the standby surgical list for the doctor was sick and planned to only take office visits that day. I returned to the treatment room and advised the Pauloses of my finding and suggested that it would be wise to perform the corrective surgery that evening as T. B. was already under sedation. They, too, felt it would be best to proceed immediately with the orthopedic surgery.

T. B. was held by Mrs. Paulos while I went out to the Mustang and brought in my anesthetic machine. While I was getting surgery ready, Mrs. Paulos explained to me what had happened. "I had gone to the grocery store and taken T. B. along for the ride. When I got home, I picked up the bag of groceries in one arm and T. B. in the other and headed for the front door. T. B. saw the neighbor's cat and jumped out of my arms injuring herself. I saw the leg was damaged and then called the hospital."

Mrs. Paulos continued, "I have never seen a cat run from T. B. Most cats are about twice her size and all they do is spit at her and arch their backs. Cats will face her at all times and simply refuse to be intimidated by such a small adversary. I think that someday she thinks a cat will run from her. That would certainly be an ego booster."

I connected the dog to the anesthetic machine and then walked to the front of the hospital to let the Pauloses out. Mr. Paulos asked, "I'll bet you don't know what T. B. stands for?" I said, "tuberculosis?" Both of them laughed. Mrs. Paulos said, "T. B. is short for Taco Bell—good name for a Mexican breed of canine." I agreed with them that it was a good explanation.

I returned to treatment and prepared T. B. for the orthopedic correction. I had selected the smallest intramedullary pin that had a threaded tip and then gloved up and went to work. The threaded portion of the pin was embedded securely in the epiphysis of the ulna. This aligned the ulna and acted as a spacer for the radius. The skin suture line was closed and I removed my gloves. I glanced at my watch and noted it was almost midnight. I now stabilized the leg to keep it in the proper healing position. A padded splint was prepared and then taped to the leg. T. B. now sported a suitable walking splint.

The anesthetic machine was disconnected and T. B. was placed in the recovery ward. His injured leg had swollen slightly due to the trauma so I injected the steroid, vetalog, to reduce it. Now it was clean-up time. The instruments were cleaned and placed in a surgical pack. I left the pack for morning sterilization then called the Paulos's house and gave them the post surgery report as I had promised. I reminded them that I would call again about seven in the morning when I rechecked T. B. The gas machine was returned to my Mustang and I headed for home. I pulled into my driveway a bit weary at one thirty that morning.

# —33—

# A SIDE STICK

I t was after supper when the call came in. The Gardena operator said that the owner had a German Shepherd that had a severely mangled rear foot that needed medical attention. "May I connect you with Mr. Stromgren?" Almost immediately I was talking to the client and agreed to meet him at the hospital.

King was able to walk into the treatment room and I assisted Mr. Stromgren in lifting King up on the exam table. King weighed ninety pounds and was a load for even the two of us. It was a large laceration and fortunately no primary vessels or nerves had been involved. Mr. Stromgren held King's right front foot while I sedated him then put him on the gas anesthetic machine. I cleaned up the lesion by debriding it and removing the hair and debris that had accumulated on the bloody surface. I told the owner what needed to be done and he wanted to remain and watch me do surgery. I explained to him that I did not need any distractions from an observer and preferred to disappear into my own world of surgery. Mr. Stromgren understood and retired to the reception room where he said that he would find a magazine to bide his time.

I completed surgery and bandaged the foot. Then I invited the owner in to see King while his pet was still on the surgery table. I thought my move was sensible for then he could help me put King in a cage in the recovery ward. When he saw King's bandaged leg, he said, "King won't keep that on long! He has been sutured before and he will certainly remove the bandage and chew out the stitches." With this in mind, I put on my thinking cap. There were no collars large enough to fit this size dog. I remembered using a side stick on a large animal when I was in school. I looked around for a broom that would soon need to be replaced and then searched for the tool box. I located a saw and and an electric drill with accompanying bits. I was in business.

I measured the distance from King's collar to midthorax and cut the broom handle about six inches longer. Then three inches from each end I drilled a hole. I used a piece of heavy cord to tie one end to King's leather collar and then I searched for something strong to put around King's chest to attach the other end of the stick. I could find nothing. Mr. Stromgren volunteered the use of his belt. This worked fine and now the broom handle was secured at each end. King now sported a side stick. This apparatus would eliminate his head and neck movement so he could not reach his hind quarters and remove the work I had spent so much time accomplishing. Now Mr. Stromgren helped me to lift King off the table and put him into the ward.

We filled out the client/patient card and, since I am so curious, I had to ask how King injured himself. Mr. Stromgren did not know. It was a mystery. He explained, "My wife won't let me smoke in the house and when I went out the backdoor to the yard, King was there with an injured foot. I thought it was more prudent at the time to see that King had medical attention than to search for the cause of his injury. In the morning when it is light, I will look around the yard for clues." As soon as the man exited the hospital, he lit up a cigarette. He was standing outside his car enjoying his smoke when I left the hospital so I walked over and visited with him before heading home.

Marna was walking in the backdoor with an armload of groceries as I pulled into the garage. I helped her carry the rest of the sacks in and put them on the kitchen counter. Marna said that she had just met a client of mine while she was standing in line at the store. "The lady in front of me was holding a Chihuahua that had a bandage on its front leg. I remarked what a cute dog it was. We chatted for a few minutes and finally got around to introducing ourselves to each other. When she heard my last name she asked if I might be the veterinarian's wife that did the surgery on T.B. I said that he had done surgery a couple of weeks ago on a Chihuahua that had jumped out of its owner's arms.

Mrs. Paulos then asked me to tell you that T. B. is now doing fine. She said, 'Cats now run from him because when he runs, the splint makes a sharp noise when it hits the ground and I think that is what scares the cats. T. B. thinks that he is now dominate and is so proud of the fact that cats are afraid of him. It sure looks funny to see a three pound dog chase a ten pound cat.'" Marna and I both laughed at the scenario as we put the groceries away.

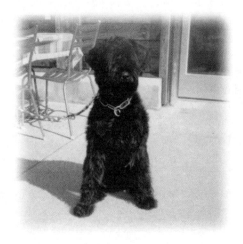

# —34—

# MY INTERPRETER

Allen was now in his sophomore year in high school and taking his third year of German. He was in his room studying when I asked him to assist me. The Torrance operator had connected me to a client that she had difficulty understanding. I, too, faced the same problem but recognized that she was speaking with a prominent German accent.

Allen took the receiver from me and soon was involved with the lady on the other end of the line. I could not understand what the conversation was but noted that Allen nodded on occasion and shook his head at other times. I interpreted these actions as positive and negative but there were gaps in between that were unknown to me.

Finally he put his hand over the receiver and turned to me saying that Mrs. Straubing was on the line. Her cat had a swelling at the base of its tail, and could I see her this evening? I confirmed that I could and I would meet her at the Torrance hospital in thirty minutes. Allen relayed this information and an appointment was made. I asked Allen to join me.

Allen and I arrived first and opened up the hospital. We visited for several minutes before Mrs. Straubing arrived with her domestic male cat named Bach. He was a five-year-old male and solid black in color. Bach had a pronounced swelling at his tail head. Allen filled out the client/patient card for me and we proceeded into the examination room. Bach's temperature was slightly over 103 degrees indicating a fever. I parted his fur and found two teeth marks about one half an inch apart in the affected area. A cat bite abscess was now the confirmed diagnosis. I discussed with the owner through Allen what needed to be done. She desired to wait until the abscess was lanced and then go home after she saw Bach's surgery was completed. Allen suggested that she return to the waiting room. He then carried Bach into the treatment room. I corrected him for referring to the front room in that manner and suggested that "reception room" sounded better. He agreed with me.

It was good to have experienced help, and in no time at all Bach was lying relaxed on the table after receiving the surital. The abscess was lanced and both Allen and I curled up our noses as the putrid fluid was expelled. The pocket that contained the purulent matter was lavaged first with a sterile saline and then swabbed with an antiseptic solution. A seton drain was established to keep the wound open so it could be treated for several days.

As a cage was prepared for Bach, Allen went to the reception room and invited Mrs. Straubing back to check on her pet before she left for home. When she entered the treatment room, she remarked about the foul odor. We had forgotten to warn her about the smell as we had become insensitive to it as we worked on her pet. Allen explained to her that Bach would get a medicated bath in the morning to remove any of the stench that may linger on his fur. He directed her to call in the morning for an update and to find out the time of discharge as well as to set up an appointment in four to five days to remove the seton.

Mrs. Straubing remarked that she had married a serviceman about three years ago. She had been raised in Bavaria and was learning to perfect her English. She thanked Allen for being knowledgeable in German and said that he spoke better German than she did English. This brought a smile to Allen's face.

It was still relatively early in the evening so we stopped and got some ice cream and chocolate sauce. Allen also selected some walnuts and a few bananas. Marna fixed sundaes for the boys right away. Marna and I decided to partake of ours later.

While Allen indulged in his ice cream, he explained what he had said to Mrs. Straubing in German. He could not think of what a seton was called and had to use the word "drain" instead. I assured him that it was an adequate synonym. The two youngest settled down for the night and Allen continued with his studies.

Later Marna and I relaxed in comfortable chairs in the family room to enjoy our ice cream sundaes. We were both tired from our day's activities and were just glad to sit and visit. The quiet of the evening was interrupted by the sound of the telephone ringing. The answering service for Redondo Beach was on the line and they wanted to patch me into the dispatch switchboard of the Redondo Beach Police Department. The switchboard would relay the message from Sergeant Gilbert of that city's K-9 unit. Nikki, the police K-9, had an injured shoulder that needed medical attention. We agreed to meet at my own hospital in Redondo Beach in twenty minutes. I hurriedly finished my ice-cream sundae, followed that with a swallow of coffee, and was on my way.

I pulled into my hospital parking lot and the police car with a huge K-9 emblem on the side of it was already waiting. I introduced myself to Sergeant Gilbert and he in turn introduced me to Nikki who was on a leash. Nikki was a six-year-old male Rottweiler and a beautiful dog. We proceeded into the reception room as I held the front door open. As Nikki passed me I noted a gash on his shoulder that had stopped bleeding. A lot of dried blood was matted to the hair beneath the lesion.

I filled out the patient card and escorted the law enforcement team to the back of the hospital. The sergeant put Nikki up on the treatment table. Now the lesion was more closely inspected. It was a clean cut about five inches long that would require suturing. Sergeant Gilbert held Nikki securely while I close clipped the area around the lesion and cleaned up the blood that had dried beneath the wound. I painted the area with a surgical prep solution. The officer thought I could probably apply the sutures without administering any anesthetic so I commenced. However, every time I would attempt to place the needle through Nikki's skin, he would twitch his shoulder muscles and shy away from me. The officer knew I was having difficulty performing my task but still did not want me to give Nikki a general anesthetic. I suggested a local anesthetic as an alternative. He readily agreed.

I infiltered the area around the lesion with xylocaine and waited about five minutes for it to take effect. It was now easy to apply the fifteen or so sutures as Nikki felt no discomfort and stood stock-still while I performed my task. I gave an injection of an antibiotic and told the officer that surgery was over and he could lift Nikki off of the table. He noted the tub in the grooming room nearby and asked if he could put Nikki in the tub and give him a quick bath and towel-down. I obliged. Nikki was soon on the floor again, ready for action.

I inquired as to what had caused Nikki's injury. Sergeant Gilbert said, "The doctor's office nearby has a silent alarm and the security company responded to it. When they pulled in, the security guard noticed a flash-light beam playing across the wall from the outside window. He notified our department and asked for assistance. Two cars responded—my K-9 unit and another patrol car. We surrounded the building and ordered the intruder out. No response. We again used the megaphone and still no response. We could find no place where the intruder gained entry so we called dispatch and asked them to phone the owner so he could come down and unlock the front door instead of us trying to break in. Shortly the doctor arrived. He stood carefully to one side as I unlocked the glass door. We swung the door open wide and again repeated to the person inside to come out with his hands on his head. There was still no response.

"One of my fellow officers turned off the electrical power at the meter. I shouted that the power was off and I was sending in a dog. I released Nikki and instructed him to 'search.' Within two minutes, Nikki barked and then a male voice was shouting, 'Call off you dog, I'm coming out.' Nikki had him cornered and he was afraid to move.

"The electricity was turned back on and we entered and found Nikki still holding this man at bay. The man was still clenching a plastic bag and pharmaceuticals were scattered all over the place. A chair was turned over and blood spots were on the floor. I initially thought that Nikki had grabbed the man, but the perpetrator denied that he was bitten. I then noticed that it was Nikki that was bleeding.

"We cuffed the man and escorted him outside. We asked him what had happened and he said that he had tried to fend off the dog with the chair but couldn't see well in the dark. He said that he was very scared of the dog. We put the man into the other patrol car for his voyage to the booking center. I then called you to get my K-9 taken care of."

Fortunately it was only a skin wound and I told him that it would heal well. It really didn't seem to bother the dog. The sergeant said, "Nikki will be able to complete his patrol duty tonight so he will not be able to draw any of his sick leave."

I suggested that the stitches stay in for ten to fourteen days and Sergeant Gilbert said that he would remove them himself. He paid Nikki's account in cash and requested a receipt so he could be reimbursed by the city. The sergeant and Nikki returned to duty, and I returned home.

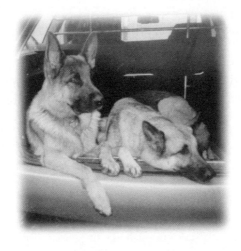

# 35—

# July 4th Hysteria

**I**t was the Fourth of July and I had spent considerable time on the phone all day as well as the night before. Everyone wanted advice on how to cope with their pets' adverse reaction to the noise of fireworks. Mr. McCarthy wanted to meet me at the Gardena hospital and get some more tranquilizers. Beebe needed some help as she was terrified and the medication that they had been giving her apparently was not strong enough to have the desired effect. Mr. McCarthy seemed really stressed and I agreed to refill the same medication that had already been prescribed but if a new medication was to be dispensed, I would need to see the patient.

Marna needed to stay home and relay emergency calls to me. The neighbors invited my three sons to go with them down to King Harbor and watch the City of Redondo Beach's fireworks display. The neighbors picked the boys up just as I was leaving. We headed in opposite directions.

Mr. McCarthy and Beebe were both anxiously awaiting my arrival. I unlocked the front door and pulled their card from the files. I assumed that I might be prescribing a different medication since Beebe was present. "Doc," Mr. McCarthy said, "It's pretty quiet down here and my wife and I thought it would probably be better for all of us if we just boarded her here at the hospital for the rest of the day and pick her up sometime tomorrow. Beebe is completely uncontrollable at home. When fireworks started going off late this afternoon, she hid in my son's room

150

and chewed up his teddy bear and then destroyed the bedspread. We scolded Beebe and confined her to the garage. While in jail there, she would bark and whine. When we went out to admonish her, she had obliterated a sleeping bag we had stored there and trashed my gardening gloves. We just don't have any quiet place for her away from the noise. Can we kennel her here?"

I assured Mr. McCarthy that we had room in the boarding ward so I prepared a cage and then asked him to lead Beebe into the ward and place her on the towels that I had used to pad the cage.

The owner left and I called to check with Marna about any other emergencies that may be on my agenda. There were none so I returned to the ward to put a pan of water in Beebe's cage. The towels that had been her bed were in shreds. One fragment of the terry cloth towel was hanging from her mouth.

I made a bed for her in an adjacent cage. I could not hear any outside noises from the fireworks but I knew that canines have a keener sense of hearing than humans so I gave my nervous patient an injection of a tranquilizer and hoped that she would calm down and rest comfortably for the remainder of the holiday. I trashed the scraps of towels from her previous cage and headed home.

It was about two in the morning when I received my third call of the night. The Manhattan Beach operator had a Mrs. Putnam on the line concerning her coughing dog, Trixie. "Doctor, Trixie has been coughing a lot the past day or two but tonight it is much worse. It is so bad that she is keeping both my husband and I awake. Fred insists that I call you or put Trixie in the garage for the rest of the night. I guess that means I will have to take her to the hospital."

I soon had Trixie, a female silver Poodle, on the exam table and was taking her temperature. There was a significant fever. Her chest was clear. My examination using the stethoscope was only interrupted by her persistent coughing. No wonder no one in her household could get any sleep! I opened her mouth to examine the tonsillar area, but my line of vision was impaired by saliva and foam. In order to accomplish a more thorough exam, I felt that it would be necessary to sedate my patient.

Foam was swabbed from the throat. Both of her tonsils were enlarged and protruding from their tonsillar crypts. I did not suspect a foxtail or the like hidden in the tonsillar crypt as the inflammation was bilateral, but strange things do happen, so a careful probing was done. No foreign body was discovered. I gave Trixie a steroid injection to reduce the inflamed tonsils and an antibiotic to decrease her fever. Mrs. Putnam wanted to know what needed to be done next.

I explained that Trixie had severe tonsillitis and if the injections did not reduce the size of the tonsils, the doctor in the morning might recommend a tonsillectomy. That decision would be entirely up to him.

"What made him cough so much?" she asked.

"When the tonsils become so enlarged that they bulge out of their tonsillar crypts, Trixie thinks that she has something in her throat and tries to cough it up. Unfortunately this irritates the tonsils even more so the condition progressively becomes worse. I think that was Trixie's problem. What caused the original irritation is a guess."

I put Trixie in a cage and when we checked on her later, she was standing up and poking her nose through the bars on the cage door. I brought her out to the exam room and gave her a hycodan tablet that contains codeine to reduce her coughing reflex. I found some honey in the refrigerator and mixed a teaspoon of it with a small amount of warm water. Then I put the mixture into a squeeze bottle and squirted some into Trixie's mouth. This would give her some comfort from the irritated throat that she was experiencing.

I indicated that Trixie could go home now and that Mrs. Putnam could either make an appointment for tomorrow now or she could phone in the morning and make one then. "Doctor, I think it would be best to leave her here for if she coughs any more and disturbs Fred, he will be upset. I think leaving her is the best decision."

I located the patient card in the files and filled in the pertinent data. After Mrs. Putnam left, I attached an additional note to relay the emotions of the evening and advised the doctor to phone me at my hospital if he had any questions. I left a note on the cage for the staff not to feed Trixie for she might be a surgery patient.

# 36

# FIREWOOD

Allen and George watch M.A.S.H. on television and get into the habit of using the word "stat" (meaning "right now") in our household. I cautioned them about using that word when they asked their mother to do something for them. But like all children, caution was thrown to the wind. When I got home from my evening emergency, Albert was playing in the family room and Allen and George had each been confined to their individual rooms.

I asked Marna what had happened and she said to ask Allen and George. I went into George's room and sat down on the edge of his bed to hear his story. George said, "Mom asked if we would like a cup of hot chocolate. Allen said, 'Yes' and I said 'stat.' Mom didn't appreciate my remark and when we both started laughing, she got upset and sent us to our rooms." I wanted to laugh, too, at Albert's story, but restrained myself. Next I went to Allen's room and heard the same story. He was upset because George had said "stat" and caused all of the problem. He said, "All I did was laugh!"

I went back out to Marna and she was laughing now, too. At the time of the disturbance, she was busy fixing dinner and doing laundry and just didn't take kindly to the boy's demanding tone when she was only trying to be nice to them. We were interrupted by the telephone. Mr. Laughton had called through the San Pedro exchange. His German Shepherd, King, had injured its mouth, and he surmised that some dental work would be necessary. I agreed to meet him at the hospital in about an hour.

Mr. Laughton had King on a leash in the parking lot when I arrived. King was drooling bloody saliva when we went into the treatment room. I checked his mouth and one of his upper canine teeth was missing and the other upper one was very loose. His lower canine teeth were attached more securely but were bleeding around the gums.

"I have never seen this type of injury before," I remarked.

"It is unlikely that you will see another one of this nature either," responded Mr. Laughton.

"What happened?"

"I have about two acres of avocado trees in the hills and since I have retired, those trees occupy most of my time. I have a pickup and King rides in the rear. King has the habit of collecting wood and whenever I stop around the orchard, King jumps out and searches for a piece of wood. If he can pick it up he carries it to the truck and deposits it in the pickup bed. I got back to the truck early and whistled for King. He came running with a piece of an old fence post in his mouth about three inches in diameter and maybe two feet long in his mouth. I get tired of having to continuously dump wood out of the truck, so I thought I would teach him a lesson and started back to the house in a hurry without him.

"King saw me leave and decided to take a shortcut. He tried to run between a tree and a post that were barely wide enough to permit him passage. I looked in my rearview mirror and saw my dog flying through the air. He landed in a heap and just lay there. I thought he had broken his neck. I circled back and parked next to him. He was moving so I rationalized that he had only been stunned. It was hard work to lift a limp ninety-pound dog onto the truck bed. When I got to the house, I left him in the truck while I went into the house to call you. I returned to the truck only to find King at the back door waiting for me. His mouth was partially open and he was drooling."

I told Mr. Laughton that we had better take an X ray to see if any serious damage had occurred. No fractures were noted. I then gave King a short acting anesthetic and extracted the other upper canine tooth that was malaligned and very loose by now. I checked the rest of his mouth and all I could determine that was wrong was the two lower canines that would move slightly when I applied pressure to them. They needed to be protected if they were to be salvaged. I recommended that King not chew on anything hard for a couple of weeks to give those teeth in question a chance to stabilize.

"Doc, that will be hard to do."

I asked if there was a place where King could be confined.

"Yes, but when I do he barks and annoys my neighbors. He is especially noisy when I go in my truck and leave him because he likes to ride with me everywhere."

I decided to send home some tranquilizers to keep him quiet. I told Mr. Laughton, "If they don't do the job, come back in for a refill. Stronger medication can be sent home if necessary. Also a soft food diet is a necessity."

"All he eats is dry food, Doc."

"Soak it in some gravy, meat essence, or water and let it stand before offering it to him. From the looks of King, I don't think he has missed very many meals so he should readily accept it."

"I understand. I am really glad you didn't say any longer. You know, King has probably collected enough firewood to last all winter. Most of it is the proper length and only on occasion do I have to cut any of it. It is interesting because when I empty the wood from the truck, I throw it into a pile by my storage shed. He never bothers it again. He only loads my truck with wood he scavengers from other places on the premises. We will have to wait and see if this escapade will convince him that what he is doing can be dangerous."

I noted that King was coming out of surgery rather quickly, so Mr. Laughton and I slid King over on a gurney and rolled it out to the truck. We then put him onto the bed and Mr. Laughton headed for home. I hoped that King would not wake up sufficiently before he arrived there.

# -37-

# A PILLOWCASE CARRIER

**A** light rain was falling. Marna had changed into her robe and slip-pers, and we were enjoying the fire in the family room as we each held a cup of hot spiced apple cider. The aroma of cinnamon permeated the room. We were just relaxing and enjoying the quiet of the evening when the silence was suddenly interrupted by the sound of the phone.

The Torrance exchange connected me with Mrs. Filbert who wanted assurance that the problem with Cassy, her cat, could wait until her regular veterinarian's hospital opened the following Monday morning. Cassy had some scabs on her head and ears and was paying considerable attention to that location. She would take several steps, then stop and scratch at them with her rear feet. "Is there anything I can do to help relieve her of this discomfort until Monday morning?"

I was not any more eager to go out that evening than Mrs. Filbert was, so I suggested that she wrap Cassy's rear feet in masking tape so her claws would not scarify her head and ears. This will frequently discourage a cat from scratching near their head since the noise of the masking tape rubbing against their scalp annoys them. Mrs. Filbert said that she would comply with my suggestion and take Cassy into her regular veterinarian first thing Monday morning.

Marna and I had just finished our second cup of cider and I was banking the fire when the phone rang. It was Mrs. Filbert calling back. My suggestion had worked fine—for ten minutes. That was about how long it

156

took Cassy to remove the masking tape. "I think the tape on her feet bothered her more than the scabs on her head. When the tape was removed, she returned to her original problem of scratching her head. Now there are places on her head and her left ear that were bleeding. Can you see Cassy tonight? She shakes her head and flings blood around so I have her confined to the bathroom where it is easy to clean up." I told her that I could leave right away and asked her how long it would take her to reach the hospital.

"I don't have a cat carrier and I don't want blood all over my car. What do you recommend I do?"

I suggested that Cassy be put into a pillowcase and then tie the top so she couldn't escape.

"Won't she suffocate?"

"No," I answered, "She should transport very well and be in no danger."

I took off my slippers and put on a pair of shoes, picked up my waterproof jacket, and was soon on my way. I arrived at the hospital, opened up, and waited. And I waited. Twenty minutes had elapsed past our agreed upon meeting time and still no owner or feline in sight. I obtained her phone number from the answering service and called her directly.

"I am waiting for you at the Torrance hospital," was my first comment.

"Doctor," she said, "Have you ever tried to stuff a frightened cat into a pillowcase? I am scratched up and there are blood spots over the bathroom walls and fixtures. I am a nervous wreck, and Cassy is as scared as all get out!"

I was amused at her comment and understood her predicament. "Let's try a different approach. Let Cassy calm down for a minute or two and then put the pillowcase over her when she is either standing or sitting. When this is accomplished, flip the pillowcase so that it trips her then tie the top."

"Do you really think it will work?"

"I have done it that way before, and it is certainly worth a try. I'll stay on the line until you have Cassy confined in the case."

A few moments passed before Mrs. Filbert retunred to the phone. "It worked, doctor, she is now in the pillowcase and crying incessantly. I will leave immediately."

Shortly a car pulled into the parking lot and Mrs. Filbert and a vociferous Cassy arrived. Cassy, a calico female, was very happy when I took her out of the pillowcase and placed her on the exam table. Her right ear had been scarified and a couple of spots were now noticeable on her head between her ears. No bleeding was evident at this time for she had been unable to scratch at her ears from the confines of the case. However, once on the table, she was showing signs of a severe pruritus and the itching and scratching syndrome was again initiated.

The entire top of Cassy's head as well as the external parts of her ears showed signs of hair loss and were covered with crusty scabs. I was immediately suspicious of mange. I related to Mrs. Filbert what my suspicions were. She couldn't believe that was possible as her two other cats had no evidence of this problem. I got permission to do a skin scraping. I placed the skin scraping on a glass slide and used a glass cover slip. The specimen was scanned under the microscope and no mites were found. I picked another location and repeated the procedure. The results were again negative.

Mrs. Filbert was becoming a bit impatient. I returned to the exam room to take my third sample. Mrs. Filbert said, "Is this really necessary?" I assured her that it was and explained that the mites are sometimes very hard to locate.

I treated the third scraping as I had its predecessors. Mrs. Filbert was standing first on one foot and then the other as I used the microscope again to scan the sample. I was relieved when I located two active sarcoptic mange mites in the same field. I returned to the examination room and restrained Cassy while Mrs. Filbert took a peek through the microscope at my findings.

"What causes the intense itching?"

I responded by saying, "The movement of the mites and their secretions and excretions."

"What next?"

"A lime sulfur bath works best. Cats are not usually dipped but they are allowed to soak in the solution for at least twenty minutes until it dries on them. Then they are confined to a cage for about a day. I must warn you. They take on a characteristic yellow color that stains their coat and may last as long as two or three weeks. This treatment is effective, however."

"When will the treatment be done?"

I checked the hospital and located the lime sulfur solution. "I can do it tonight and Cassy can probably be picked up the day after tomorrow."

"That would be fine," she said. "What about my other two cats?"

"If they are not showing any symptoms now, no treatment needs to be initiated immediately, but I think for prophylaxis that I would certainly have the other two cats treated in the same manner. They have been exposed if they have been together and the likelihood of being infected by the mites is great. The best thing to do is to talk it over with your regular doctor when you pick up Cassy."

I again reminded the owner that Cassy would be so yellow both on her skin and coat that she might appear jaundiced. I put my patient into the bathing tub and then located an old smock and put an apron on over it. I almost forgot to don long-sleeved rubber gloves. Soon I was properly attired and ready to go to work. Cassy was a bright yellow when she had finished soaking and I put her into her cage. I headed for home after being gone almost three hours.

It had been raining off and on for the past several days, and the clouds had decided to open up in earnest. I was experiencing a downpour as I pulled into my garage. When it rains in this manner, few calls usually come in. This is not uncommon because pets stay close to home or within the house where it is warm and dry and are not exposed to the many hazards of life. However, Mother Nature has her own schedule, and the Reeses were on the Palos Verdes line concerning Lucy who was in the first stages of whelping. She was straining a lot but so far had been unable to deliver any of the pups. I agreed to meet them at the hospital within half an hour. Allen had just finished his studying and had come out into the kitchen in search of a snack. I asked him to join me and we were soon heading west toward the coast.

Both Mr. and Mrs. Reese were taken into the treatment room where almost everything I would need to assist Lucy was handy. Lucy was a three-year-old Malamute and a beautiful dog. She was registered and had been bred to a registered champion. Four of the pups had already been spoken for and any more than that could easily be sold.

I could palpate five fetuses in her abdomen. I gloved up and checked to see if she had dilated. She was well dilated but no fetus was in the birth canal. I slowly administered the hormone oxytocin intravenously. In about three minutes Lucy started straining and was in active labor. Mr. Reese held Lucy's head and within minutes I was holding the first pup in my hands. I opened the amniotic sack and clamped off the umbilicus with a hemostat and handed the pup to Allen. Allen wiped the mucous from the pup's mouth and helped it obtain its first breath of air. The Reeses had used some foresight and brought with them a wicker basket with a folded blanket in its bottom. Pups were arriving in a rapid fashion. When each pup was breathing, Allen handed the pup to Mrs. Reese with the hemostat still attached to the umbilicus and she would dry it off and place it in the basket. This procedure was repeated until the basket contained six crying and active Malamute pups—one more that I could identify by palpation.

When Lucy was completed with her labor, Allen would retrieve a pup at a time and I would tie off the umbilical cord with suture material and release the forceps. The Reeses were delighted. Only four pups had been spoken for and now they had two more to sell. When Allen returned the last pup to the basket, he announced, "Three males, three females."

The Reeses took care of their account and departed. Allen and I turned to the chore of restoring the place to order. Before we walked out the door, the phone rang and I had an emergency at my hospital in Redondo Beach. We headed north for about a mile in the slackening rain.

The Gilbertsons arrived shortly with Dagma, their chocolate Labrador. Dagma was vomiting. In fact, Dagma had not kept anything down for almost twenty-four hours. The Gilbertsons said that he had ingested some baked potatoes that had been wrapped in foil. Some pieces of the foil had been identified in his vomit. With this information in mind, I prepared the X-ray room to take a couple of lateral views of Dagma's abdomen. Pieces of foil were noted in his bowel but none appeared significant enough to cause a blockage. I discussed this with the owners and recommended a barium series to see if the radiograph would indicate where the problem might be located.

There was a definite blockage in the small intestine. None of the barium sulfate had passed that specific location even after four consecutive views taken at fifteen minute intervals. Whatever caused the blockage was not visible on the film but it was evident that the object had formed a dam and not allowed any of the barium media to pass that point. The Gilbertsons and I were puzzled what caused the problem but agreed that a laparotomy, an investigative surgery, was necessary.

Allen brought in the anesthetic machine, and I prepared for surgery. The Gilbertsons held Dagma in the reception room until I was ready for my patient. Allen then brought him back again to the treatment room where I soon had Dagma resting easily after inhaling some of the metafane gas. The Gilbertsons decided to wait until the puzzle of the blockage was resolved so they returned to the reception room. Allen and I prepared Dagma for investigative surgery. It did not take me long to locate the problem. I could palpate the bowel and soon located a structure within its lumen almost three inches long and about the size of a small broom handle. I proceeded with an enterotomy and removed a cork. I closed the incision and soon Allen disconnected the anesthetic machine and rolled it out to the Mustang. When he returned, he brought the Gilbertsons back and I showed them what I had retrieved.

Mr. Gilbertson's story was fairly complicated. "Two nights ago we invited a couple over to our house for dinner and bridge. We had stacked the dishes on the kitchen counter and retired to the bridge table. Dagma was in the house because of the rain and while we were engrossed in the card game, he became a kitchen scavenger. He is big enough to stand on his hind legs and devour any leftovers on plates left on the counter. This included the remains of foil wrapped baked potatoes and anything else that smelled good. The cork was from our wine bottle and I just didn't think of that when we talked earlier."

Dagma was resting well and would be hospitalized for two days depending on his progress. They left the required deposit and were about to leave when I asked them the origin of Dagmar's name. "I assume it is a Swedish or a Scandinavian name and if so, what does it mean?" Both of the owners laughed and said that question is frequently asked of them especially since their name is of Swedish origin. Mrs. Gilbertson said, "Dagma is an acronym. When we got the dog, we could not decide on a name. There are five persons in our family and we had that many sugges- tions. Each one of us insisted that our name selection was superior to the others. I decided on a ballot and I asked each member of the family to put down their initials when they returned the ballot. Two days later I had all five ballots in my hand. The solution was still not resolved. While the children were touting their own selection, I started looking at their initials. I then combined them into Dagma. 'D' is for Dad, 'A' is for Anne, 'G' is for Geoff, 'M' is for mother, and 'A' is for Alice. We took another ballot after I explained what my selection stood for and the vote was three out of five. Dagma became his name. In answer to your question about the meaning of his name, my answer is none."

Allen helped me put Dagma in a recovery cage and we then headed for home. Allen wanted to stop for a late snack but we put that idea on hold when the rain began coming down in earnest again. As I stepped into the house, Marna handed me the phone. I was able to answer all of the client's questions and assure her that her pet was not in immediate danger and could wait until her regular doctor was on duty to care for her pet.

It was late the next morning when I had a phone call from the hospital where I had treated Cassy the night before. The attending doctor said that Mrs. Filbert was aghast at Cassy's yellow color. The doctor related that, "She knew his coat would be yellow but did not realize that it would be such an intense color. I sent home a cardboard carrying container to transport Cassy in and to bring back her other two cats for the lime sulfur treatment. I just did a skin scraping on her black cat and found sarcoptic mites on my first try. Now Mrs. Filbert will have a herd of bright yellow cats at home until the color wears off."

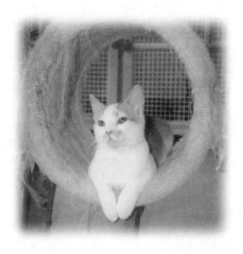

# -38-

# TRAPPED IN A TRENCH

**M**ark O'Neil, the husband of one of Marna's friends, called me at home Saturday afternoon. Chester, their mixed black and tan terrier, was missing. What should be done? His dog had dug a hole under the fence sometime the night before and had escaped. "We have looked everywhere for him. We posted lost dog signs all over the neighborhood and have received no response. Do you have any suggestions?"

I certainly had not had any emergency Friday night concerning a dog of that description. I suggested that he check with the lost and found editor of the local newspaper. There were also several hospitals in the area that I did not have under contract for emergency care and I gave Mark their names so he could contact them. "I will call around to see if I can be of any help, and if I get any information at all, I will let you know."

I had admitted a surgery case over the weekend at my own hospital. This meant that I had surgery to do before I commenced taking appointments for the day. I arrived at my hospital early and there was a car waiting in the parking lot. It was Mark O'Neil with Chester. He followed me into the hospital and I pointed to the exam room. I then took off my coat and put on a smock before joining them.

Chester had been lost all weekend. Mark said, "A construction company had been installing a large sewer pipe in their neighborhood and somehow Chester had fallen into the trench and could not get out. We had looked for him there on Sunday, but he must have walked into the large pipe and couldn't hear us when we called for him. When the workers arrived early this morning, they found Chester in the trench. They lifted him out and gave him to a nearby resident. Everyone seemed to know who Chester belonged to since we had not only posted signs, but we had talked to numerous people and knocked on many doors as well."

"He looks pretty good to me," I said.

"I think so, too, but he is limping on his right front leg and that seems to bother him." I checked the leg but could not elicit any pain. We took him into the X-ray room and in a few minutes we were both scanning the wet film together. "I still can't find anything wrong," I said.

I palpated the leg again manipulating it carefully. No response was noted until I hyperextended the leg. When I did this he attempted to retract his foot from my grasp. It bothered him but he was not complaining very much. I placed him on the floor again and he still exhibited the mild limp. "I think that Chester overextended his elbow when he fell into the trench."

"Can you give him something for pain?"

"I don't think he is in severe discomfort and I would prefer not to give him any medication. Anytime he overuses his leg and feels a twinge of pain, he will be reminded to be more cautious. Remember, we cannot communicate with pets like we do people. They are not capable of under-standing logical reasoning so discomfort provides a limiting factor in their aftercare." I did give Chester a cortisone injection and enough of the medication in tablet form for three days.

Mark told me that he had one happy family when they got a call that Chester had been found. His wife stopped by the donut shop and got a dozen donuts for the construction workers as a thank you for finding Chester.

I had heard of a Jack Russell Terrier, I had read about them, and I had looked at pictures of them, but I had never seen one until now. I was at the Hermosa Beach hospital, looking at Carson, a member of that breed. The Brackets were across the exam table holding their pet. Carson was in distress. He was slightly dehydrated and was standing in such a manner that indicated to me that he was uncomfortable and probably hurting internally to some degree. The Brackets told me that he had not eaten for two days but appeared to be thirsty. However, he would drink and then a short time later would vomit up the fluid. They could not think of anything that Carson might have consumed that could cause the symptoms that they had been describing to me.

I could not palpate anything identifiable in his abdomen that would indicate a blockage of his intestinal tract. When I again checked his abdomen, I located a firmness in the small intestine about six to eight inches long. I surmised that it was related to an obstipation. To confirm this, I advised the Brackets that I should do a barium study of the gastrointestinal track and proceeded when they replied in the affirmative.

Carson was anesthetized and connected to the gas machine. I passed a stomach tube and deposited some barium sulfate into his stomach after first taking an initial reference view. Every ten minutes another view was taken as we followed the passage of the barium media through the stomach into the small intestine. When we looked at the third film, I noted a distinct change in the flow of the media. Only a thin thread of the media was now appearing in the lumen of the bowel. Something that was not delineated by X ray was impeding the passage of solids and only allowing a minute portion to travel through the bowel at that location.

I advised the Brackets of a blockage in the small intestine and received approval to proceed with a laparotomy. Carson was prepared for surgery after the owners decided to return home. I locked them out and returned to surgery. A ventral midline incision was made in the abdominal wall. I located the portion in question and reflected it out of the body cavity where I could evaluate the problem more astutely. It reminded me of pajamas or a swimming suit that had been gathered up with a string or cord. I could feel a small lineal object that appeared to traverse the area in question. I then made a small enterotomy incision in the middle of the puckered area and exposed a piece of string. Now I had located the cause of Carson's problem and proceeded to remove it.

The anterior portion of the bowel was milked away from the incision until all of the gathers were gone and the bowel was straight. Then by holding the bowel so that it would not pucker up again, I applied gentile tension to the string and was able to pull that end of it through the small incision site. The same procedure was used on the distal portion and all went well. Soon I was able to display a piece of stout string about a foot long on my mayo tray. All had been recovered via a half-inch incision through the intestinal wall.

I closed the bowel incision, then the skin incision, wrapped a bandage around Carson's middle, and disconnected the gas anesthetic. I fixed a cage for my patient and cleaned up surgery before calling the Brackets because I wanted Carson to show some kind of alertness before I gave a post surgery report.

The Brackets must have been waiting for my phone call because they picked up the phone instantly. I assured them that Carson was doing fine and shared with them my findings. They had no idea where or when Carson had ingested the piece of string. I suggested that it may have come off of a tied meat roast, but they ruled that out because they were vegetarians. The cause of the emergency remained a mystery.

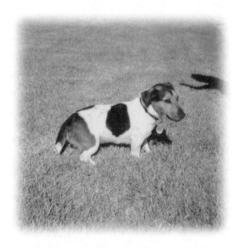

# — 39 —

# MY CALL FOR HELP

I t was late on Saturday afternoon and my emergencies at the Hawthorne hospital were stacking up. One case was already on my surgery agenda and two cases to be examined were waiting in the reception room. I had just hung up the phone after asking another client to come to the office in approximately twenty minutes.

I needed help, so I called Marna to have her bring Allen down to assist me. I was in the examination room with my second client when my son arrived. Marna stayed for awhile and helped too until I was caught up with all of the pets that required immediate attention. Marna took control of the front desk, and Allen became my helper in both the exam and treatment rooms.

The second and third cases involved dogs with an allergic response and a foxtail in the ear, respectively. They were treated and dispatched. The case that was in transit had just arrived and before Marna had a chance to pull the client's card from the files, a lady came in with a dog cradled in her arms that had just lost a race with an automobile. Marna hustled the accident case immediately into the treatment room and I excused myself from the waiting client that I had just invited into the exam room and proceeded to the rear of the hospital.

The client that was just getting up to bring her pet into the exam room said, "I was next!" Marna tried to explain that I was attending a more critical case and would be with her shortly. Marna said, "If the situation was reversed, how would you like to be treated?" Shortly the accident case was stabilized, and Allen was keeping it under observation. I returned to the exam room to take care of my disturbed client. As soon as I entered the exam room, the client apologized for her unnecessary remark to Marna. I accepted her apology and explained that it is always necessary to practice triage when dealing with emergency cases and that means treating the most critical patient first.

While I was with Mrs. Curry and Bum in the exam room, Marna admitted a cat belonging to the White family that had a nasty looking abscess on the side of its neck. The tiger-striped cat named Mandy had had abscesses before, so the owner, Mrs. White, knew what to expect and left Mandy in our care.

Mrs. Curry held Bum, her mixed terrier, while I examined a cut on his shoulder. It would require suturing and I recommended she pick her pet up in the morning when I had to come in and do treatments. I caged Bum and now I had the accident case on the treatment table and two surgeries on hold.

A mild sedative was administered via the intravenous setup that had earlier been connected to the accident case. Allen and I then took Bennie, a Beagle male, into the X-ray room. Bennie had multiple fractures. A severe fracture of the pelvis, a pelvic symphysis separation, and a green stick fracture of the left femur were very evident on the film. Allen helped me put a temporary splint on the leg and then we carefully placed Bennie in a well-padded cage in presurgery with the intravenous drip still connected.

Allen brought Bum out and he was sedated. Allen clipped the hair from his shoulder and then scrubbed around the wound and painted it with an antiseptic. In a few minutes I had the wound closed with sutures and Bum was returned to his cage.

Mandy was brought out and the abscess was lanced under sedation and treated as needed. Since I planned to discharge her in the morning when I came in for treatments, I asked Allen to give her a bath now to save time on Sunday morning. Now I had time to pay more attention to Bennie who was beginning to respond to our treatment and show some signs of life. We jointly carried Bennie back out to surgery dragging the intravenous setup behind us. He appeared alert now and over the critical aspects of shock. The pelvic fracture involved the ilium that was separated and out of line. The gas machine was connected to him via an endotracheal tube and his hip was prepared for surgery. Using two

Steinmann pins, the ilium was aligned properly and stabilized in that position. Since Bennie was still under the effects of the gas, I refashioned the temporary splint. Allen disconnected the Beagle and we placed him in recovery.

I was busy filling out the patient records and bringing all of them up to date on the cases I had attended to that afternoon when Marna returned to the hospital with soft drinks and sandwiches. She had stepped out unnoticed and gone down to the corner fast-food establishment to get all of us a treat.

I called the Curry house and brought them up to date on Bum. When he was waking up, he had vomited all over himself. Allen had put him into the tub so he would be nice and clean and smell good when he was discharged.

All three of us worked to put the hospital back in proper order. It was now time to go home. Marna said that she had spent so much time helping me that she had not had a chance to start supper. In fact she had not decided what to fix. I suggested that she pick up George and Albert and meet us at one of the boys' favorite restaurants—one that made delicious hamburgers. I called the answering services and gave them my forthcoming location and telephone number. Allen and I then departed. All three of the boys were delighted about the suggestion of eating out. We had a leisurely meal of shakes and burgers, and to make the outing perfect, I had no telephone interruptions.

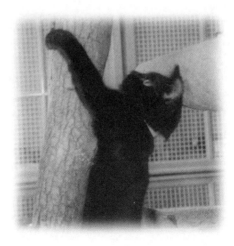

# —40—

## JUST DO IT!

**A** misty rain was again falling over the South Bay and gradually saturating the area. It was more of a nuisance type of rain than a soaking rain for it did not come down hard enough to wash away the road scum and dirt. All it did was streak windows and cars and draw attention to the need for them to be washed. I was standing on the front porch wondering if the rain would stop or commence in earnest when the phone rang. I disengaged myself from the sweet aroma of falling rain and went inside to pick up the telephone.

The Torrance exchange informed me that Mrs. Olivet was on the line and only wanted to ask me a few questions. I was quickly patched through. Bonnie, her Golden Retriever, had been brought home from the hospital this morning. Bonnie had been spayed and now she had chewed out three or maybe four of her sutures. I explained that this was an outer layer of sutures and that another row of sutures was underneath the visible skin sutures. This reassured her to some degree.

"What happens if she chews out all of these stitches?" she asked.

"The skin sutures can be replaced in the morning if you take Bonnie back to your doctor. The important thing is that you will have to put a wrap on her belly to discourage her from removing any more of the stitches. Do you have an Ace bandage or some other type of bandage in your house?"

"Yes, I have saved the bandage my daughter used when she sprained her ankle."

170

"Place some gauze over the incision site and then put the bandage over it and wrap it completely around her body. Next take some adhesive tape or, if none is available, use masking tape and cover the bandage with that. Hopefully that should deter her from paying any further attention to her surgery."

"Thank you, doctor, I will do as you suggested."

Later that night I had a return call from Mrs. Olivet concerning Bonnie. Bonnie was paying attention to her spay incision again. I listened to Mrs. Olivet as she said, "Bonnie, somehow, has nosed the bandage aside and chewed out more sutures. I am really concerned. It looks worse than before and I think a piece of her bowel is now bulging out. I would feel much better if I could bring her in and have you take a look. I really would sleep much better tonight if you would just take a peek at her and reassure me that no problem existed."

I agreed to meet her at the Torrance hospital in half an hour. She arrived with her daughter shortly after I opened the hospital. Mrs. Olivet was calm and collected but her ten-year-old daughter, Beth, was crying and carrying on to such a degree that Bonnie was becoming hard to manage and somewhat protective of Beth.

We went into the exam room. I excused myself because I wanted to locate the client/patient card, but it was hard to find because it had not yet been refiled. Beth remained in a chair in the reception room and was still crying. Bonnie was on a leash and wanted to inspect her surgical site again but Mrs. Olivet would give the leash a tug each time and this distracted my patient from doing any further damage.

We lifted Bonnie up on the exam table and rolled her over on her side. The bandage was in disarray and upon careful examination I noted that several sutures on the inner layer had also been chewed out. No intestine was visible but it was very possible that an evisceration had occurred. The bowel may have been exposed for a short time and had fallen back into the abdominal cavity when we had turned her upside down. Bonnie was put under anesthetic and four deep sutures were replaced first and then the skin layer was resutured. I put a secure roller gauze wrap around her body and then covered that with two layers of four-inch elastic adhesive tape. Now she had the appearance of a dog wearing a girdle.

The Olivets had waited during surgery. Beth had composed herself and I was now able to communicate with her and reassure her that Bonnie would be okay. They had a good look at Bonnie, and Beth patted her as I disconnected the anesthetic machine. I picked Bonnie up, carried her in to the recovery ward, and placed her in one of the lower large cages. Mrs. Olivet was concerned that when Bonnie woke up, she would again commence to chew at the stitches. I comforted both of the ladies when I brought in a plastic collar, and with Beth holding up Bonnie's head, I positioned it around the retriever's neck and snapped it in place. Then I demonstrated how Bonnie could not reach her ventral midline as long as she wore the collar.

They had numerous questions about her aftercare that I answered as best I could but I suggested that they ultimately discuss Bonnie's surgery and the problems she had had with their doctor when she was discharged in the morning. I received a thank you from Mrs. Olivet and a tearful smile from Beth. Before they left, Mrs. Olivet told me, "Bonnie is really Beth's dog. Bonnie had belonged to my mother and just before Mom died, she asked Beth to take care of Bonnie for her. Beth assumed the responsibility and the two are now practically inseparable."

Most of the time emergencies are spaced out so I can care for one patient without interruptions. My next emergency came in from the Manhattan Beach hospital about eleven in the evening. The next emergency I received was less than a minute after I had hung up the phone. Fortunately, the first phone call seemed to be the most urgent so I responded accordingly. I met Mr. Pelton at the hospital and he brought in Fargo, a male apricot Pug, for me to see. Fargo had been stepped on and he was carrying his front paw. It was painful when I rotated one of his toes and I could feel crepitation when it was so maneuvered. X rays needed to be taken, and when I told the Peltons that Fargo would stay the night and go home in the morning, they readily agreed and left for home.

I injected a sedative in the muscle and put him in a cage temporarily and headed for Gardena for my second emergency. The client, Mrs. Whitmore, had only been waiting a few minutes. She brought in Motley, her five-year-old male cat, who had an eye problem. Motley had a prolapsed right eye.

"This is a serious problem," I said. "Why didn't you give me some clue over the phone how bad it was?"

"I didn't want to look at it because I have a very weak stomach and didn't want to get sick. Besides I couldn't get here any faster as I had to get dressed. I only had to wait a couple of minutes so really no time was lost."

I checked Motley more carefully and noted that his front claws were frayed. "How long ago do you think this might have happened?"

"Not more than two hours because when I let him out, he was not injured," was her response.

"The eye needs to be replaced in the socket." I glanced at Mrs. Whitmore. She was pale. Motley was put in a cage in a hurry and I ushered Mrs. Whitmore out to the reception room and seated her before getting her a glass of water.

It took a few moments for Mrs. Whitmore to adjust to the situation. Finally she said, "Don't tell me what needs to be done—just do it! Cost is not an issue." I tried to explain that Motley might lose vision in that eye, but she raised her hand to stop my conversation. "I'll rely on your professional judgment to do your best surgery and take care of Motley so please don't say anything more. I don't want to pass out."

I asked her if she was feeling better and she said, "Good enough to drive home." I assisted her out to her car and she thanked me and left. I administered a light sedative in one of Motley's muscles and then a stronger one in the vein in order to pass an endotracheal tube so I could perform surgery when he was under the anesthetic. The right eye had prolapsed because of a sharp blow to the head. Gently the eye was replaced in the socket and the eyelids were sutured together. Next a compress was placed over the eye and then securely taped in place to insure that the replaced eye had sufficient pressure on it at all times. Motley was placed in a cage before I headed back to Manhattan Beach to check on my first patient, Fargo.

Fargo did not know when I arrived or how long I had been gone because he was still under the influence of the sedative I had given. I used a short-acting anesthetic in his vein to insure the proper level of narcosis to allow me to treat his foot properly. An X ray was taken and the radiograph indicated that one of his metacarpal bones was separated by a fracture, and an adjacent one sported a very evident hairline fracture. I injected a steroid to reduce the swelling and went to work.

I taped the two fractured toes to the ones on either side. Then I fashioned a walking splint on the foot so there would not be any movement of the toes if he became too active. Bones will not heal unless they are held immobile. I then called the Peltons and gave them a progress report. They thanked me for keeping them informed and said they would call in the morning when the hospital opened.

Everything was put away and I headed back to Gardena to see how Motley was doing. Motley was raising his head slightly and then plopping it down when he got tired. This was repeated two or three times before I was able to provide a better cushion under his head. I did not want the jarring action of banging his head down to cause any further damage to his injured eye. I had left the surgery room in a mess when I had departed so I cleaned it up and filled out the patient card. I left an inconspicuous note telling them where I had left the two one hundred dollar bills that Mrs. Whitmore had left for a deposit. I mentioned on the card that Mrs. Whitmore was very sensitive to any surgery details. I climbed into my Mustang and pointed it south toward home.

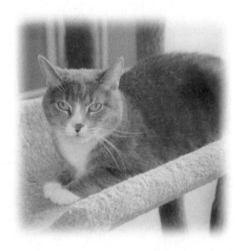

# —41—

# A TRANSFUSION

The Lawndale exchange was on the line when I got home from work. As I was talking to the operator, I could see Marna making me a sack dinner. She could sense from my conversation that I would not be home to enjoy dinner with my family.

The operator connected me to the McKeevers. Scotty, their Scottish Terrier, had just been hit by a car and was in critical shape. He needed attention as soon as possible. I agreed to meet the family at the Lawndale hospital and left immediately, grabbing my sack dinner as I passed the kitchen counter on my way out.

I had to compete with rush-hour traffic but soon I arrived at the hospital and found the McKeevers anxiously waiting. We went into the treatment room immediately and Scotty was placed on the table. He was comatose and had difficulty breathing. I was able to insert an endotracheal tube and connect him to oxygen without sedation. His shallow respirations improved slightly.

Blood was being discharged from the edges of his mouth and this indicated the possibility of internal injuries. A plasma expander was started in his vein, and saline and dextrose with solu-delta-cortef was injected into the intravenous tubing. Scotty's breathing was gradually improving and becoming more regular. I wanted to give a unit of whole blood but there was none on hand at the hospital. I called around and located some at an El Segundo hospital and asked Mr. McKeever if he would pick it up while

175

I attended to his injured pet. He said that he would be happy to oblige and was on his way. Mrs. McKeever and her two young sons stayed and helped me monitor Scotty.

Mrs. McKeever was a very capable assistant and I remarked how efficient she was. She said, "I was trained as a nurse but haven't practiced nursing since my first child was born." She was more than willing to help me in any manner and I took advantage of her skills.

Scotty was now blinking his eyes—his only movement noted so far other than his breathing. He groaned slightly when I straightened his legs to a more suitable position. Mr. McKeever returned with the unit of blood and I connected it on the other front leg with another intravenous set. We slid Scotty off onto a gurney and rolled him into the X-ray room. Several views of his chest and abdomen were taken and Mrs. McKeever and I reviewed them together. Mr. McKeever had retired to the reception room to be with his sons. I could hear him reading a story to the boys.

The radiographs revealed a fracture of the left humerus near the shoulder and three fractured ribs on the same side as well. The diaphragm was still intact and very little fluid had accumulated in either his thoracic or abdominal cavities. The fractured edges of the ribs may have indirectly accounted for the bloody discharge from his mouth. My first responsibility was to stabilize Scotty. Shock was a major concern and he appeared to be responding well to treatment. Mrs. McKeever proved to be a great assistant.

Finally she said, "Is there any coffee in this place?" I directed her to where it was located and she disappeared. Ten minutes later she handed me a cup of steaming coffee. I asked her to take a cup out to her husband. "I've already done that and I fixed some of that instant cocoa that was on the shelf for Kent and Kerry. Hope that was alright?"

Scotty had been badly shaken up. He had certainly received a severe blow. The wheel of the car must have hit him on his left shoulder to cause the damage that we were now evaluating. Mrs. McKeever had seen the accident and said that that was exactly what happened. "We were taking the boys to soccer practice and put Scotty out in the backyard. The side gate must have been left unlatched for when we started down the street we noticed in our rearview mirror that Scotty was chasing after our car. We had traveled only a short distance and pulled over to the side of the road to allow him to get into our car. That is when he was hit by another car.

"Scotty was hit solidly and spun around and ended up near the curb. The driver of the car felt terrible but explained that he never saw the dog. It was not his fault. We put Scotty on the back seat and went home and called our hospital and they contacted you."

I suggested they take the boys home. It had been a rather traumatic evening for them and they needed to be home in their own surroundings and relax. All four of the McKeevers left for home. I poured another cup of coffee and sat down with my sack dinner.

Scotty was continually showing signs of improvement and that was very encouraging. I was trying to decide if it was time to move him to one of the cages in the critical care ward when there was a knock on the front door. Mrs. McKeever had returned to help me. Mrs. McKeever was able to locate a large beach towel. She then rolled it up sideways and laid it next to Scotty. We rolled our patient up and over the roll, flattened the towel and tilted him back into the same position he was previously. I had never done this on pets before—probably because it is a two person procedure.

We rolled the gurney and the intravenous stands into critical care and then raised our patient up by lifting the towel with our little black dog in it. He was gently placed in the cage and the tubing was organized so it would not crimp if he moved.

We enjoyed another cup of coffee before she left for home. I stayed until a little past midnight. Scotty was trying to lift his head now. The unit of blood had been given and the plasma expander was almost gone. The accompanying saline and dextrose drip was slowed down so it would last until the morning staff arrived to take over. The patient card was completed and it was now time for me to journey home as well.

# 42 —

## ANOTHER CALL FOR HELP

**M**arna and I were outside walking around our yard and, in a sense, "smelling the roses." It was spring and most of the flowers that had been planted and cared for were exhibiting their beauty and fragrance for both man and bees to enjoy. When the yard is inspected, there is always a list of little things noted that require attention. Marna stood beside me with a pad and pencil making notes. We returned to the garage and located a basket, gloves, and the necessary tools to accomplish the tasks before us. I heard the phone ringing and went inside to answer it.

The Hawthorne exchange was calling in regards to a Dachshund that was owned by the Kingmans. I was patched through to the owners. "Robby had been out in the yard and when he came back inside, he was dragging his rear end," was the complaint.

I changed out of my gardening clothes and was soon heading north on Crenshaw Boulevard. I was just about to the railroad crossing when the safety barriers came down and the lights started flashing. A slow freight train was soon creeping by. I thought it would take an eternity to make the crossing before the barrier would be raised and I could be on my way. About the time I felt the endless train would clear the road, it stopped and slowly began to back up. I turned off the engine and waited. Twelve minutes later the road was clear and the traffic that had collected was allowed to move. Now I had congested traffic to contend with. It took me forty-five minutes to reach my destination.

Both Mr. and Mrs. Kingman were impatiently waiting but understood the delay when I explained the circumstances. Robby was checked and I explained what I thought the problem was—a herniated disc. If corrective surgery needed to be done, time was a factor. I was not skilled in this type of surgery so I planned to call a veterinarian in the west Los Angeles area to seek his advice.

Several X rays had been taken before I sought council with Clayton, and while we were on the phone, I was looking at the radiographs in the viewer. Two discs in Robby's back were involved for they had prolapsed and were infringing on the spinal cord. Clayton said that he would like to talk to the clients.

After an extended conversation, I was handed the phone. Clayton said, "They have agreed to both the surgery and my fee. I have my sterile surgical pack in my car and should be at the Hawthorne hospital in twenty-five to thirty minutes. Get surgery ready and have the Doxi under anesthetic and prepped for a hemilaminectomy when I arrive. This will cut down considerable time, and time is an essential factor in repairing this type of injury."

Clayton arrived and we went immediately into surgery. The Kingmans planned to leave and go out to dinner and return afterwards. I acted more like an anesthesiologist than an assistant surgeon as I watched Clayton's skilled hands manipulate the discs in question. Soon he had completed his portion of surgery and I was allowed to do the skin closure. Clayton and I were reviewing the surgery, and I had many questions for him regarding his technique. The Kingmans had not returned from dinner and Clayton wanted to discuss the aftercare directly with them to avoid any misunderstanding that might possibly occur.

I was cleaning up surgery and visiting with Clayton when the returning owners knocked on the front door. Clayton met them and we all sat out in the reception room and discussed the case and its forthcoming care. Clayton wisely brought a printed handout that he uses to emphasize the care in post-operative cases. He carefully went over all of the details with the Kingmans. I was impressed with his thorough approach. Robby was to be confined at the hospital for several days, so we took them back to see their reclining pet and then they departed for home.

Clayton said that he hadn't eaten since breakfast and was starving. He suggested that we go out to dinner. I called Marna and told her where we planned to dine so she would be able to forward any calls to me. Clayton did not have a hospital of his own and, in a sense, was a contract veterinarian like myself. I contracted for emergencies while he did only specialized surgeries. He said that my business card should read, "Have car will travel" while his should say, "Have surgery pack will travel."

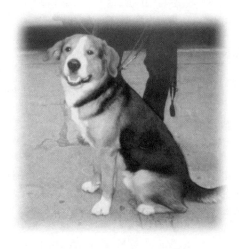

# —43—

# A CAR, A BIKE, A DOG

**I** was just walking out of my hospital after a busy day. Jo had some bookkeeping to do and she did not want to carry that over into the next month so she was busy with pencil and calculator as I left for home. The parking lot was as far as I got when a car with a bike stuffed in the trunk pulled into the driveway. Ted Alton stepped out of the passenger side and came over to my Mustang.

"Glad to catch you, doc, before you left," was his initial remark. "Genny is injured and needs to be checked over!"

I pulled back into my parking space and told Ted to bring in his dog. Jo had recognized him and already pulled his card. Genny was a female Boxer and had been involved in a traffic snarl. The gentleman who had been driving the new Lincoln had followed us both into the hospital. He told Jo that he would cover all expenses and handed her his credit card to record. He asked her to fill it in after all costs were calculated.

The Boxer was left with us and the gentleman said that he would take Ted home and then Ted could return in his own car. Ted asked me to wait for him. He said that he would be back in about twenty minutes. I checked Genny over. She had numerous road burns as well as a laceration on the side of her neck that would require sutures to close it. I did not perceive any reason to take radiographs so Jo held Genny and I gave her some surital in the vein to relax her in preparation for surgery. Jo did the clipping and I applied the antiseptic solution, cleansed the

181

wound, and then closed the tissue with sutures. We had just completed the surgery when Ted returned. I now noticed that he had a skinned elbow and a torn shirt as well as several grease stains on his trousers. He said that he and Genny had been involved in a minor traffic accident.

Ted said, "Since I retired, I spend a lot of my time on my bicycle down at the beach. I was peddling along and a girl walked by. I glanced over my shoulder to get a second look and in so doing I swerved the bicycle out into the traffic lane. Genny was on a lead and running along beside me. Needless to say, I swerved at the wrong time. Mr. Abrams sideswiped me. I ricocheted to my right into a parked car. Genny was caught between the bicycle and that car and got injured. Mr. Abrams was very concerned for both Genny and myself. He offered to drive me to the hospital but I assured him I was only scratched up. The front tire of my bicycle had buckled so he offered to take me home. I was more concerned about Genny and he said we could drop her off at my regular veterinary hospital first. Now I am here for my second visit of the day."

I walked him back to see Genny on the surgery table and he gave her a pat before we took her into the recovery ward. Ted said that he would call me in the morning. He left and Jo noted that he drove a bright red Porsche. Jo later said that Mr. Abrams was certainly a nice man to go out of his way to assist Mr. Alton. She said, "Somewhere during Mr. Alton's conversation, I heard him say that he was retired. He must be in his early thirties and that is kind of early to retire, isn't it?" I told Jo that he was one of those wiz kids who had formed a company before he was twenty-five. Two years ago he sold the business for several million dollars. All he does now is enjoy life by spending most of his time on a bicycle or on a surf-board. I was surprised that he allowed Mr. Abrams to pay for the veterinary services when I know that he has plenty of money. After looking at the car Mr. Abrams drove and at Ted's Porsche, I don't think either one of them is hurting for funds.

Later that night a client of mine was on the phone. The answering service had alerted me to the fact that all three of the Spencer's pets were sick to their stomachs and had been vomiting since about noon. I was connected to Mr. Spencer a few minutes after I arrived home.

When he got home from work, his dogs Blue and Spot, as well as his cat Tiger, had been sick to their stomachs since late morning. Blue, a male

Australian Shepherd, was the only pet that still showed some of the symptoms. Spot, a female short-hair terrier mix, seemed to be over the problem but would not eat and was happy to just lie down in the backyard and not move about. Tiger, a male cat, had followed Spot's attitude and just lay around and wouldn't eat either. "Do you think I should bring all of them in for you to see this evening?"

I decided to ask more questions and asked, "What do you think happened? It must have been something all three were exposed to."

"I have no idea. They each eat out of their own dishes and do not scavenge from each other's food or raid the garbage can."

"Have you put out any snail bait or the like?"

"No, but I got up early and sprayed the yard for insects and then fertilized using a liquid spray. I kept the animals inside while I was doing this and didn't let them out until I left for work."

"What product did you use?"

He got out the container and read the warning label. It said that digestive upsets were possible if sprayed on animals. I reminded him that we had a lot of dew in our area this morning and asked him if they had dew on the ground where he lived. He said yes.

"I think that it is likely that your three pets got some on their coats when you let them out into the yard. If the vegetation was still wet and your three pets walked through it, some of the chemicals probably adhered to their coats. Then the chemicals were either absorbed through their skin or ingested if they had a tendency to lick themselves."

"Gosh, that is entirely possible. I never gave that a thought. I only knew that I could not leave them in the house. My wife left before I did and if I let the pets stay inside, they would tear up the place."

"I think the problem has been diagnosed. Tiger and Spot are both shorthaired. Blue has a long coat and may have had more exposure. Feed them a mixture of cottage cheese and rice and embellish it with a little ground low-fat meat. I don't think any of them could or would ingest enough to poison themselves with this type of minimal exposure but it certainly could make them sick. Try that at home first and then call back about eleven. If that doesn't seem to help, I will see your pets then."

"I'll try that. Thanks a million!"

Mr. Spencer called back on schedule and said that Spot and Tiger had eaten some of their food and appeared much better. Blue was still moping around and refused to get up and either look or smell the food in his dish at all.

Twenty minutes later I was looking at Blue who had been placed upon the exam table. I could smell something on his coat. Mr. Spencer had been around the odor so long that he was now insensitive to the smell. Blue had a normal temperature but exhibited an unnatural stance due to abdominal discomfort. I passed a stomach tube and pumped in an ounce of Mylanta. Then I told Mr. Spencer that I was going to give his dog a bath and keep him for the night. I completed the bath about half past midnight and headed home. In the morning Blue looked much better. He ate some canned lamb mixed with cottage cheese. He smelled better, too. I called the Spencer house to report on Blue's progress and got no answer. Both of the Spencers were probably at work. About an hour later, Mrs. Spencer called and I told her that Blue was doing well and she could pick him up on her way home from work.

Jo was standing in the doorway as I hung up the phone. She informed me that Mr. Alton was waiting in the reception room to talk to me before I released Genny. I told him that Mr. Abrams had called earlier to see how Genny had fared during the night. Ted said, "You just don't meet a person like that very often and when you do it is quite by 'accident'!"

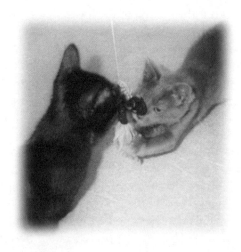

# —44—

# A CHANGE OF HEART

The hot temperature had not let up and it had peaked about three in the afternoon when I received a call at my hospital from the police switchboard in Redondo Beach. An officer had been called to a shopping center parking lot from a concerned citizen about two dogs that had been locked in a car. The officer said that both dogs were under considerable stress and that he planned to break the car's window and bring the heat-stressed dogs to my hospital. I told him that I would be waiting for him.

I prepared for two heat stroke patients. I had Jo go across the street to the liquor store and get four bags of crushed ice. A few minutes after she returned, the patrol car arrived with two limp Llasso Apso dogs. I took both of the dogs into the critical care ward and placed them in separate cages with a bag of crushed ice on either side of their abdomens. Then Jo wet terry cloth towels in cold water and placed them over the dogs' bodies and the ice bags as well. Then we used portable cage fans on each cage door to give us additional cooling effect for our comatose patients. I instructed Jo to keep the two under constant observation and to take their temperatures every five minutes for I did not want their body temperatures to go from hyperthermia to hypothermia.

The officer left his name and also the citation number that he had issued to the car owner. Another police car had been called to stand guard over the auto that the policeman had broken into to insure that no one would steal anything. Also the guarding officer would inform the owner, when he or she returned, where the dogs had been taken to be hospitalized.

Between Jo and I, one of us was monitoring the heat stroke patients at all times. I would watch when a client came in or when Jo answered the phone. Then Jo would take over when I entered the exam room to care for a patient. Three office visits later a lady who identified herself as Miss Harrison burst into the hospital. She was very upset because the police had broken into her car, removed her pets, and issued her a citation. She said that the citation for inhumane care of animals she held in her hand should identify her as the owner of her two Llasso Apso dogs. She said, "I left two windows down an inch so air could circulate but it got too hot inside anyway!"

Jo stepped out front where I was talking to Miss Harrison and beck-oned to me. She whispered to me that she thought that the older dog had just died. In the meantime, Miss Harrison tried to circumvent Jo in the hallway and go back and locate her dogs. Jo did not yield an inch and blocked the owner's way. I tried to talk to her and, after listening to some abusive language, decided to have her follow me back and show her the two dogs. On the way Miss Harrison remarked, "How dare those officers break into my car. I know how to care for my pets!"

We walked into the ward. Both of her dogs were lying there very quietly. She said, "Gracie isn't breathing!" I informed her that her older dog had just died of heat stroke. Miss Harrison just stood there with her mouth open. Finally she said, "Are you just going to stand there and let Fonzie die too?" I was more irritated than ever and said, "Young lady, I am doing all I can. Why don't you assume some responsibility for what happened and not blame everyone else for your misfortune."

After this remark of mine, she opened the cage door, I guess to take Fonzie home. She removed the towel and pushed aside the ice packs. That was as far as she got before she burst into tears. She put her hands over her face, left the hospital, and ran to her car.

We had not obtained any information from her other than the dogs' names—Gracie, the older dog, and Fonzie, the surviving younger dog. We identified Gracie as a female and Fonzie as a male Llasso Apso. I asked Jo to call the local police department and get the address and if possible the telephone number of Miss Harrison. They gave us the address that they had tracked down from the car's license plate and they called back later and gave us the telephone number that they had also been able to find.

Gracie had indeed died and I was in a quandary as to what to do. I called the police department back and they advised me to retain Gracie in the freezer I had for that purpose. Fonzi was doing better. He had lapped some water from the pan Jo held in front of him. Both Jo and I stayed until almost six o'clock. Fonzi was now standing, his temperature was normal, and he was making a feeble attempt to wag his tail.

I phoned Miss Harrison and she wanted to come right down and see her dog. We went to the back of the hospital and she opened Fonzie's cage and cuddled him in her arms. She then informed me that she was taking Fonzi home. I had already filled out the patient card and recorded the fees so I assured her that it would be fine. I handed the card to Jo and set about cleaning up the cage. Jo came back and said, "You know what happened? Miss Harrison walked straight out the front door and never even made an attempt to take care of her account!" Jo said that she appeared to be a very bitter woman.

I called the police department and related to them what had happened. They asked me what the charges were and then said for me not to worry. (I had dismissed the case from my mind until two months later when I received a check in the mail from the court. Miss Harrison had pleaded no contest to animal abuse charges. A fine had been levied that covered my fee as well.)

The day was still hot even as the sun settled over the Pacific Ocean and there was no relief from the high temperature. The one hundred degree weather was unusual for the South Bay and it seemed to wilt everyone—including Marna and myself. Once the intense rays of the sun were muted, both Marna and I sought refuge in the backyard. It was time to sit back and enjoy a glass of iced tea and recharge our energy reserves. My relaxing time on the lounge chair changed when the phone rang. Marna looked at me and that was a signal that it was my turn to get up. The Torrance exchange had Mrs. Billsley on the line and I was patched through.

The Billsley Dalmatian, Speckles, had a very sore rear end. A large swelling had developed just to the right side of her anus and it made her very uncomfortable. "It hurts her so much that when she is sitting she puts most of her weight on her left side. My husband and I just noticed it and we would like to have her attended to this evening." We agreed to meet at the hospital right away.

Mrs. Billsley arrived quickly accompanied by her niece, Shelby, who was visiting them. Shelly was twelve years old and had insisted on coming along as she had aspirations of pursuing the field of veterinary medicine in college and wanted to be an observer. When I glanced at Speckles, I saw that she had a typical anal gland abscess. I escorted the entourage directly into the treatment room and lifted Speckles up on the table to get a closer look at the problem. To the right side of her anus was a large soft swelling. I discussed what needed to be done. I asked Mrs. Billsley to hold her dog while I administered some surital intravenously to sedate her. I then asked both the mother and niece to wait in the reception room while I lanced the abscess. Shelby wanted to stay and watch but I discouraged her. Mrs. Billsley was more than willing to exit the room.

I treated the anal abscess in a similar manner as a cat bite abscess except that, since I was dealing with glandular tissue, it was necessary to cannulate the anal gland duct. I filled a syringe with sterile water and placed an adapted cannula [small tube] on it and cleared the duct. Antibiotics were given and I invited the owner and Shelby to take a look at Speckles before I put her into a recovery cage.

When they entered the treatment room they both remarked about the awful lingering odor. I had forgotten to warn them of the pungent smell. They stood at a distance as I showed them the surgery that I had just completed and how it would be necessary to treat Speckles at home after she was discharged in the morning.

Shelby looked up at her aunt and said, "I don't think that I want to be a veterinarian after all." Mrs. Billsley explained the problem by saying, "Shelby, it is just like taking care of a baby. It is more fun to feed them and clean their faces that it is to clean up the mess they leave in their diapers." I couldn't help but smile at the comparison.

I carried Speckles into recovery and placed her in a cage. I asked Shelby if she wanted to pat her before they left. She just shook her head and watched from a distance. We went to the front desk where I obtained a deposit. Mrs. Billsley said that this problem had happened once before just a few weeks prior to their move from Ohio. "Do you think this might happen again?"

I explained that it could but thought it would be best for her to discuss it with her regular doctor when Speckles was discharged.

"What causes this type of abscess anyway?"

I explained that an infection occurs in the anal gland. The glandular exudate sometimes thickens and cannot pass through the duct or the duct gets irritated and swells and thus narrows, inhibiting the passage of exudate. In either case the exudate cannot be expelled and since it is a gland, it continues to produce matter. Swelling will continue until it is corrected.

"Are these glands really necessary?"

"No, not really," was my answer. "Their primary function is to act more or less like a scent gland. When a dog defecates it exudes a small portion of the anal gland contents with their stool. As the stool passes out through the anus, the gland is squeezed against the pelvic bone. This is why dogs frequently go around and smell other dog's stools so they can find out if Spot, Ruff, or Rusty had been there."

Shelby stood beside her aunt and just listened. I never found out if she chose to pursue veterinary medicine in college.

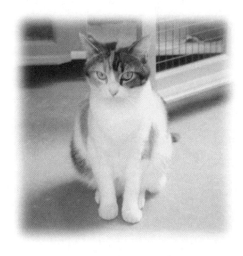

# ⌐45⌐

## CHASED BY A WAGON

**I** arrived home late because of a last minute surgery that couldn't be postponed until the next day. Marna had already fed the boys and had waited to eat until I could join her. We sat down together in the kitchen and were reminiscing about our day's events when our conversation was interrupted by the ring of the phone.

The La Rues's dog, Jingles, a Border Collie and Labrador mixture, had sustained several injuries while playing. The injury occurred a couple of hours ago but Mrs. La Rue had not phoned until her husband got home from work with the family automobile. "He feels, as I do, that Jingles's injuries are severe enough to have attention this evening." I agreed to meet them in half an hour at the Hermosa Beach hospital.

I asked Allen to go with me but that thought was negated by Marna who informed me that he had a math test the following day. With this in mind, I headed out alone. Mr. La Rue was pulling into the parking lot just as I arrived. He carried Jingles into the hospital and followed me into the treatment room as I directed. He placed Jingles on the table with the laceration on his dog's rump facing me. The lesion had been bleeding but had stopped. Jingles was also favoring his right rear leg, which was on the same side as the skin wound. I decided to take an X ray first for if I had to repair the leg, the laceration could be sutured under the same anesthetic.

Jingles was easy enough to handle and I was able to position him without sedation. X rays were taken first of the upper leg and then of the

190

knee. There was a density in the stifle joint and this indicated the possibility of an anterior cruciate ligament (ACL) tear. I manipulated the joint and the lower portion below the stifle moved in such a manner that supported the findings in the X ray. Surgery needed to be done if the leg was to be completely functional again.

The hospital's regular veterinarian did not do orthopedic surgeries and I explained this to Mr. La Rue. It would be more economical to repair the ACL and suture the skin lesion at the same time. He said that that made sense and I told him I would repair the ligament damage as well as the laceration that evening.

"When you finish the surgeries, please call me. My son is very upset about what has happened," remarked the father.

"Just what did happen?" was my question.

"Well, I didn't see the accident and I am still trying to piece together what both my wife and son told me. Billy tied a wagon onto Jingles and used him like a horse. He then rode in the wagon. This was a lot of fun for Billy and he went up and down the street attracting a lot of attention from the other children in the neighborhood. The trip up the hill was laborious and Billy had a couple of his friends help push the wagon.

"When the crest of the grade was reached, they gave Jingles a little rest and then all three of the kids got into the wagon for the downhill trip. With the wagon going downhill, it started picking up speed and soon it was going faster than Jingles could run. The momentum of the wagon finally overran Jingles. When it hit the dog, it turned him sideways and ran over the top of him.

"None of the boys were hurt when the wagon tipped over. They got up laughing at the spill and were sorting out the harness mechanism when they realized that Jingles was injured. They could see the cut on his hip and felt that his leg was only bruised. When I got home, Jingles was still limping and both my wife and I felt he should have professional attention."

I got out a text book and showed Mr. La Rue what had happened and what needed to be done to repair the injury. He asked if that was the same type of injury that football players frequently get and I assured him that it was. We discussed the cost and the hospital stay and he wanted me to go ahead with the surgery that night. After he left, I went back to surgery and located a bone drill and a bit. Neither had been used for some time so I put them into the autoclave to sterilize while I got both the surgery room and my patient ready. Before surgery was started, I decided to call home and tell Marna that I would be home late. Jingles was anesthetized and prepped for surgery and soon I was putting on my surgical gloves and settling down for an hour or so of work.

An incision was made near the laceration and about the length of the humerus for it was my intent to graft a piece of muscle fascia to replace the ruptured tendon. The fascia strip remained attached at the stifle so that the substitute tendon would have a viable blood supply. Next the joint was exposed. Holes were drilled into the joint and out the lower section. Next the fascial strip was fitted through the two holes and snugged down to tighten the joint. The end of the strip was sutured in such a manner that the joint would remain in its secured position.

I could hear the phone ringing but just had to let it ring because I didn't want to break surgery at this stage. It did not take long to close the synovial sack of the joint which was followed by the suture line on the skin. I then moved the drape over slightly and sutured the laceration. I removed my gloves and disconnected the anesthetic. I then called Marna to see who was trying to reach me. I did not have another emergency. I had just been gone so long that Marna was concerned. I told her I would be home within the hour.

I returned to the ward and organized a cage for my patient. The leg was supported with a splint and antibiotics were given to alleviate any possibility of infection. The instruments were cleaned, put into a pack, and then autoclaved. While I was waiting for the sterilization to be completed, I returned both the treatment and surgery rooms to their original degree of cleanliness. Soon I was pulling out of the parking lot and heading for home. Marna was up waiting for me so I related the story to her about the runaway wagon.

I checked on Jingles early the next morning and he was doing fine. I left a note asking the doctor to call me. I wanted to talk to him about Jingles aftercare because there were certain instructions I wanted him to relay to the client.

# -46-

# A Fall from a Ladder

I was on my way to Hawthorne to meet Mrs. Grayson who was bringing in her dog, Wilber, who had been injured. I arrived before my client and had time to open up the hospital and pull the patient/client card before she arrived. The records indicated that Wilber was a male Welsh Terrier about six years old.

I heard a car pull in and soon Mrs. Grayson entered with the black and tan terrier in her arms. I checked Wilbur first in the exam room. He seemed bright and alert but was not inclined to move around very much. His vital signs were in the normal range, but he remained motionless and just stared at me. I placed him on the floor and then called him to come over to me—he did not move.

Wilbur was again placed on the exam table and I checked each limb and could elicit no discomfort. He reminded me of a limber statue for I could move his body parts and he allowed me that privilege. I wished that he could talk. I looked up at Mrs. Grayson and she too had that faraway look in her eyes, but I was able to communicate with her.

She said, "Wilbur and I have both gone through a very hair-raising experience. I just got back from the hospital where my husband is now. We had an accident a couple of hours ago at home. My husband has been repairing the roof on the garage by himself. He was carrying a bundle of shingles up the ladder when he slipped. He fell and dropped his load of shingles and in the melee, he pulled the ladder down with him.

"Jim is in the hospital now with a broken leg. He was my first priority. I heard the calamity from the kitchen and went outside. Wilbur and Jim were both hurt and just lying there. I lifted the ladder off Jim and pushed the shingles aside. I then took Jim to the hospital after carrying Wilbur into the garage and placing him in his bed.

"When I got back from the hospital, I checked on Wilbur. He was positioned exactly as I had left him. He would watch me, but he would not make any attempt to move. I called the exchange and was connected to you. When I picked him up to put him in the car, he did not complain.

"I am not certain that Jim knows exactly what happened because he was still in a daze when I left him. I would guess that either Jim, the bundle of shingles, or the ladder more than likely fell on Wilbur, because when Jim was up on the roof, Wilbur would patiently wait at the base of the ladder for him to come down."

With this additional information, I checked Wilbur's eyes with an ophthalmoscope to see if he may have signs of a concussion. Again, no symptoms were evident. I suggested that Wilbur should be hospitalized and kept under observation. Mrs. Grayson readily agreed that it made good sense. "I have an injured husband to care for and worry about, and Wilbur might require considerable attention that I would not be able to provide."

I said that I would watch her dog for awhile and then check on him intermittently this evening and through the night. I would also check on him in the morning on my way to work. I assured her that I would call if anything dramatic was noted. I stayed for about an hour. Wilbur remained where I had placed him in the cage; he finally lay down and watched me watching him.

When I returned later that night, Wilbur was still lying down but in a different position in the cage. He raised his head and looked at me when I entered the ward. I placed him on the treatment table and checked him again. Nothing in my examination seemed to indicate that anything was wrong. I gave him a pat and he licked my hand. Dogs in pain rarely do this so I was encouraged about his progress.

About seven the following morning, I opened the ward door. Wilbur was standing with his nose between the stainless steel cage bars and whining a welcome to me. I located a leash and snapped it on his collar. He followed me to the treatment table and I noted he had a very stiff gait. On the exam table, he was rechecked—still nothing was noted. My provisional diagnosis was that he was knocked out or stunned because of the traumatic experience and remained in a daze for awhile until he was able to regain his composure.

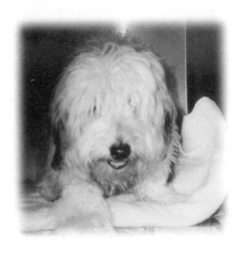

# —47—

# BASKET FULL OF PUPPIES

I had a phone call from the Hawthorne hospital asking me to take their treatment cases over the three-day Labor Day weekend. They also wanted me to cover for any cases on Saturday morning as no doctor would be present. I could not leave my own practice but promised to drop by after my hospital closed at one o'clock that afternoon if the staff would let me know if any treatment cases needed attention.

It was just past noon when Jo informed me that Hawthorne had called and wanted me to stop by on my way home. Hawthorne did not close their doors on Saturday until three in the afternoon, so I knew that some of the staff would be present to lend me a hand. The staff had several pets ready for their annual vaccines when I arrived. I was treating a cat with a skin rash when the receptionist informed me that a lady with a convulsive poodle was on the phone. I was asked if I could stay long enough to see the case. I agreed to wait. In the meantime, I went next door for a deli sandwich since a busy afternoon and holiday weekend was ahead of me.

Mrs. Mahoney arrived with Bridget, a silver poodle about three years of age. On her arm was a basket that contained five very active and healthy ten-day-old puppies. Momma dog was having tremors and could not stand. I had one of the assistants take the basket of puppies into the other room and this gave me the opportunity to diagnose Bridget's problem where she would not be concerned about her family.

All evidence indicated that Bridget had eclampsia. Eclampsia is a loss of calcium in the blood stream. The vigorous pups were removing milk from her faster that she could produce it, causing a calcium deficit in her system. I set up an intravenous drip of a calcium solution and had one of my assistants hold Bridget so she would not fall off of the table. I watched Bridget for awhile and then returned to Mrs. Mahoney and explained the treatment process and also that Bridget was showing signs of improvement. The solution would take at least an hour to administer. I informed her that it would be imperative to supplement the feeding of the pups at home or Bridget's condition would recur. The hospital stocked a supply of canned milk and some small nursing bottles. I asked the staff to set some aside to be dispensed when Bridget left for home. I encouraged Mrs. Mahoney to get the pups drinking milk out of a dish as this would make life much simpler in caring for the five little ones. One of the staff members agreed to stay past closing time to keep a watchful eye on Bridget. I said that I would return in a couple of hours and see if all was going well.

I suggested that Mrs. Mahoney should take her precious basketful of pups home with her. She said that she had an appointment on Tuesday to have the tails docked and the dewclaws removed. She wondered if it could be done a few days earlier. I had her leave the pups and told her I would call later and then she could come down and pick up Bridget and her family.

I solicited the assistance of another employee and docked the tails and removed the dewclaws. We performed this surgery in the exam room far away from Bridget so their squealing would not make her nervous. Sutures were required at all surgical locations. As soon as all five were taken care of, they snuggled back in their basket and went to sleep. I knew that they would not remain quiet long for soon their bellies would be empty and they would want to nurse. The staff agreed to feed the pups using the small nursing bottles with the appropriate sized nipples while Bridget was still connected to the drip system.

While all of this activity was in full swing, the receptionist asked me to call the San Pedro hospital. I returned the call and had a case in the harbor area that was not critical but required my presence. I left instructions with the staff and pointed my Mustang south toward San Pedro.

Mr. Oglethorpe was waiting for me with Matilda, his German Shepherd, when I arrived. Matilda was led into the hospital and I noted that she was walking very gingerly on her feet. Mr. Oglethorpe said that Matilda runs loose and somehow got into tar. "There is quite a bit of it on her feet. I got some of it off, but after awhile she would not permit me to help her any more. She wants to remove it herself. She has chewed her feet raw trying to be self sufficient and it now hurts her so much, she has difficulty walking."

Matilda would not let me touch her feet. I was able to get a cursory glance at one of them when the owner held up one of her legs. Considerable tar was noted and now I had the job of helping remove it. Removing the tar would take some time so I brought in my anesthetic machine, sedated Matilda, and inserted an endotracheal tube connecting her to the gas. She was now unconscious and I was able to get to work.

While Mr. Oglethorpe waited in the front room, I began the procedure. First, I trimmed off as much tar as possible, then I looked around the hospital for some solvent. Forty minutes later the tar had all been removed but now I had to contend not only with the damage Matilda had done by chewing on her feet but also the irritation that I had caused using the solvent. I bathed each foot with surgical soap to counter the solvent irritation and then liberally rubbed in a quantity of soothing furacin ointment. When that was done, I wrapped the feet in gauze and covered the gauze with elastic tape to hold everything in place. Injections of antibiotics and a cortisone were given to help alleviate any infection and to reduce the irritation.

I invited Mr. Oglethorpe back to inspect my completed work. I said that Matilda could go home and dispensed some furacin and bandages. I suggested that he try to keep her feet dry. I also instructed him to take the bandages off of her feet in two days. To insure that she would not pay attention to her bandaged feet, I dispensed tranquilizers for the forty-eight-hour period to be used as necessary.

Together we lifted Matilda onto a gurney and we rolled her out to his car, then deposited her on the back seat. Mr. Oglethorpe said, "I hope she leaves the bandages alone." I recommended that he give her tranquilizers as soon as the bandaged feet began to attract her attention.

I checked in with Marna and found that I had two calls. The first call was from a party that was full of questions and just needed some advice and reassurance. The second call was in Torrance, and a Springer Spaniel had an ear problem. I agreed to meet them in a half hour.

I arrived late and apologized. I felt that it was better to stop and fill the Mustang with gasoline rather than not arrive at all. The client understood. Both Mr. and Mrs. Blume brought their brown and white Springer into the exam room. Toppy was a gentle dog. The ear really bothered him. Mr. Blume volunteered to restrain him so that I would not have to administer a sedative. Using an otoscope, I soon located a foxtail and removed it with a pair of alligator forceps. I displayed it to the Blumes and then treated the ear with an ointment. I suggested that Toppy be turned around so that I could examine the opposite ear. He didn't object at all and I removed a foxtail from that ear as well.

It was now time to return to Hawthorne and check on Bridget and her family. All of the staff had gone home except one and I asked her to call Mrs. Mahoney and have her come down and pick up her canine family. When she arrived, I explained to her about feeding the puppies. Three pups had readily accepted the bottle while the other two objected to it— they preferred Momma. A syringe was sent home to deliver milk directly into the mouths of those two problem new arrivals. I reminded Mrs. Mahoney to allow the two to get a bit hungry, then to introduce the bottle. "Once they realize that if they cooperate with your persistence of feeding them in this fashion, the battle will be over."

My further instructions were to keep Bridget away from her pups. "Allow the pups to nurse late at night and then remove them. This will enable you to get some sleep. Feed the pups every four to six hours but train them to lap milk from the pan. Pan feeding must start now!"

As Mrs. Mahoney left, I told her that the sutures on the pups would dissolve in a week or ten days. She remarked, "I thought I would have a long weekend of rest, but I can see that I will be very busy. Thank goodness, I will not have to take time off from work. Hopefully I will be able to get the pups drinking milk from a pan Sunday and Monday." The phone was ringing so I let the attendant answer it as I carried the box of pups out to the car while Mrs. Mahoney carried Bridget.

When I got back to the hospital, I was informed that the Palos Verdes answering service was on the line. The operator had two incoming calls on hold. One case involved a cat with a sore eye and the other was a dog that had been in a fight. I asked the operator to tell both clients that I would be at the Palos Verdes hospital in thirty minutes and to ask the clients to come right down. Both clients were waiting when I arrived.

Mrs. Greene had a cat named Andy and I saw her first. Her client card was located and it indicated that Andy was overdue for his yearly vaccines. I reminded her of this as we stepped into the examination room. Andy insisted of making passes at me with his front claws so I bundled him up in a large towel with only his head exposed. Now I could examine his right eye without any interference. I reflected his lower lid and awns from a foxtail came into view. Soon I had removed the entire foxtail and applied ophthalmic ointment to the infected eye. Vaccines were administered and eye ointment dispensed.

My second client had a Shropshire Terrier, named Tuff Guy, who had some battle scars that needed attention. Three places on his chest and foreleg would require suturing. I explained that sedation would be required and possibly a complete anesthetic depending on how long it took to complete the suturing. I got permission to proceed.

A surital sedation was administered in Tuff Guy's vein and soon he was immobile. I hurriedly clipped the surgical sites, debrided the wounds, and then applied the necessary sutures. By the time I had finished, Tuff Guy was blinking his eyes and wondering what in the world had happened to him during his short nap. Mr. Velasquez tendered his account and Tuff Guy was carried out to the van with my help. As they left, I reminded Mr. Velasquez again that the sutures should be removed in two weeks. He waved to me as he pulled out of the driveway into the traffic.

I cleaned up the hospital before calling Marna. She asked me to call the Hermosa Beach exchange. They had been waiting for my return call and had Mrs. Bowers on the line for the second time. I was patched through for I was told that Mrs. Bowers was rather impatient and wanted to talk to me. "My Malamute is tilting his head to one side and scratching at it with his rear foot. When Freddie scratches at his ear, he whines like it hurts him a great deal. I know it is late, but can you give my dog some relief this evening? I hate to see him suffer all night and maybe even until Tuesday morning because of this long Labor Day weekend." I headed north to Hermosa Beach.

Mrs. Bowers was a few minutes behind me. I had removed her card from the files and was turning on the exam room light when she walked into the hospital with Freddie. She helped me lift this large dog up on the exam table. Freddie was too big for her to restrain properly for an ear examination so I requested permission to sedate him. Permission was granted. A sedative was administered enabling me to remove several foxtails from his affected right ear. I rolled him over to check the opposite ear and it was clean. The right ear was treated and the remainder of the antibiotic tube of ointment was sent home with the client. I glanced at my watch and it was now past midnight.

I arrived home to a quiet household. Marna had left a light on in the entryway and I turned it off before retiring for the night—or rather the morning. I got a sleepy, "Glad you are home, Honey," from Marna before I dropped off to sleep.

My sleep was interrupted about three in the morning. I assured the client that her vomiting dog was not a critical emergency but recommended that she call back in three to four hours if the problem continued.

I was up at seven and had a dish of cereal and left before anyone else arrived in the kitchen. I had four hospitals that had cases to be treated and I wanted to be there when the morning cleaning staff was present to help me with the animals.

All went well. It was past church time, so I headed for the restaurant for brunch that Marna and I had previously arranged as a meeting place for all of us. At my last hospital stop, I had called the answering services and given them the phone number of the restaurant where we planned to meet. I arrived early and told the hostess that I may have some emergency calls. She seated me and brought me a cup of coffee. I was on my second cup when the hostess said that I had a phone call. A Mrs. Carlisle was on the line and she had a dog that was bleeding badly and needed medical care immediately. I agreed to meet her at her regular hospital in Hawthorne as soon as possible. As I paid for the coffee, I told the hostess that my wife and three sons should be arriving soon and to inform them that I had received an emergency call and had to leave.

Mrs. Carlisle arrived with two neighbors—the man next door and his teenage son. She was so upset about Toro, her Cocker Spaniel, that she could not drive so she asked her neighbor to assist her. Toro was wrapped up in a blanket and the men carried the dog directly into the treatment room.

I carefully folded back the blanket and noted a massive mammary tumor. Across the anterior prominence of the tumor was a nasty laceration that was bleeding profusely. Mrs. Carlisle said, "Toro has had this tumor for some time. I didn't think it was getting any larger recently so I haven't been in any hurry to have it removed." I looked at the wound carefully and located two arteries that were spurting blood. I clamped them off with hemostats before I took time to talk to her about what needed to be done.

Before I had an opportunity to even discuss the case with her, Mrs. Carlisle wanted to know if I could remove the tumor today. I explained that it could be done and I estimated that surgery would last approximately two hours. She received my surgery quote without batting an eye. I asked her neighbor to take her home as there was no need for her to stay. I escorted them to the door and recommended that they purchase some hydrogen peroxide on the way to clean up the blood stains that were evident on both the blanket and their clothing. I returned to my patient to prepare for surgery and was interrupted by the phone.

Marna had to call three exchanges before she located me. "Should we wait at the restaurant for you to return or head home?" was her question. They had already eaten so I asked Marna to drop off either Allen or George as I needed help in the forthcoming surgery. When Marna and my sons arrived, I had already put Toro under gas anesthetic. Toro was clipped and prepped for a mastectomy. Marna couldn't believe the size of the tumor. I told her that the tumor probably touched the floor when Toro walked as it was so pendulous. Marna said, "Poor thing!"

Allen remained and we went to work. As I dissected the tumor, Allen would pressure pack the incised area with gauze and then I would either tie off the bleeding vessels or cauterize them electrically. It was almost three hours later when I removed my gloves and stepped back from the surgery table. Allen washed up and I gave him some money to get us some sandwiches and soft drinks down the street. I cleaned up surgery after putting Toro into the recovery ward.

We didn't have a chance to eat our evening meal before the phone rang again. I had an emergency at Torrance. I scheduled it for forty minutes later. We worked together cleaning up the instruments and putting them into a surgery pack for the staff to autoclave on Tuesday.

We enjoyed our sandwiches and drinks on the run. I dropped Allen off at home and then turned north to Torrance. I had two treatment cases that I needed to follow up on that evening and I got both of them treated prior to the arrival of my emergency.

It took very little time to treat this emergency case and soon I was on my way to San Pedro to follow up on my morning treatment cases there. I then headed for home. Two more emergencies interrupted my evening and I again returned home to a quiet household sometime after midnight. Monday was another day similar to Sunday. Morning and evening treatments at several hospitals were interspersed with emergency cases of several kinds in the various hospitals in the South Bay. I ate on the run at noontime and I also missed Marna's special dinner. Instead, I had a sandwich between calls. I got home at ten and was out again a bit past eleven o'clock for my final emergency of the night.

I awoke on Tuesday morning when Marna shook my shoulder and asked me if I wanted to see the boys off for their first day of school this fall. A cup of coffee enabled me to pull myself together and stumble out into the kitchen. I gave each of my sons a hug and asked them to study hard this year. Marna got a hug too, and before I left for the office, she handed me another mug of hot coffee.

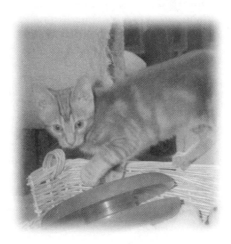

# 48

# I Didn't Mean To Do It

**B**efore I left my hospital, I had a call from the doctor at the San Pedro hospital. An emergency call had phoned in and he could not wait for it because he had an appointment that he could not miss. He said, "I still have the client on the other line. Can you take the case? If so, when will you be here?" I told the doctor that I was thirty minutes away and he relayed that to his client on the other phone line. "That will be great. Thanks for helping me out!"

I headed directly to San Pedro after asking Jo to call Marna and tell her that I was on my way to the harbor and would eat dinner later. I arrived and took the clients, Mr. Iverson and his son Tim, into the exam room with their pet, Charlie. Charlie was a mixture and it would be difficult to describe him as a progeny of any specific canine breed. Charlie's jaw hung to one side and he was drooling profusely. Mr. Iverson placed Charlie on the exam table and told me that Charlie had been hit in the head by a baseball bat.

Tim immediately responded with, "I didn't mean to do it!"

"I know son," answered his father, "I know it was an accident."

Mr. Iverson explained what had happened. "Tim was playing baseball and was at bat. Charlie got hit on the side of his face by a backswing. He went on by saying, "Tim was looking at the pitcher and didn't know Charlie was behind him. Charlie is very attentive when a ball is thrown and likes to get near the action. This time Charlie got too close."

I checked Charlie's mandible. It was broken on the right side and correction needed to be implemented soon. I suggested that surgery be done right away because their dog could neither eat nor drink in this injured condition. Besides that, Charlie was ten years old and the longer we waited to repair the fracture, the more stress it would be on Charlie. Mr. Iverson said that they would leave Charlie in my care and call the hospital in the morning. Tim was in tears, hanging his head down and blaming himself for Charlie's misfortune. I looked at Mr. Iverson and suggested that a stop at the ice cream parlor down the street might cheer up Tim.

They left after I had asked their assistance in holding Charlie while I administered the intravenous anesthetic. I walked out with them to retrieve my anesthetic machine from my car. I locked the hospital door and returned to treatment where Charlie was now located. I intubated him and clipped the fur around his lower jaw. The X rays that I had previously taken were placed on the view screen to assist me in the surgical repair. The radiograph indicated a relatively clean fracture with few bone fragments present.

I selected the proper intramedullary bone pin before putting on my surgical gloves and starting surgery. The two pieces of the mandible were united properly. I moved Charlie's jaw up and down a few times to be certain it articulated properly and conformed to the opposing maxilla, or upper jaw. The excess portion of the pin was cut off so Charlie would be able to eat and drink. I was now done.

Charlie was placed in a recovery ward cage. I decided to call the Iverson household and talk to Tim. I assured Tim that Charlie would heal alright and he would go home in a day or two. I was on my way home after cleaning the instruments and returning the premise to its normal state of cleanliness. When I got home and walked into the kitchen, Marna was on the phone. As soon as she saw me, she handed me the phone across the counter. The Manhattan Beach exchange had a Mrs. Thompson on the line concerning her pet poodle, Silver.

"Silver is unable to urinate and is very uncomfortable. My husband checked him and felt a large mass in his tummy area and thinks he may have cancer. Can we make an appointment for first thing in the morning or should he be seen tonight?" I explained that I felt the situation was critical enough to warrant seeing Silver right away. We agreed to meet at the hospital and I left immediately.

I was waiting for them. They exclaimed, "You must be a new doctor here. We have never seen you before." I explained that I only took after-hour emergency cases here, but I had been providing that service for almost six years. We went into the exam room after I had located the client/patient card from the files.

Silver was definitely uncomfortable. His temperature was normal and his coloring good. I turned him around to palpate his abdomen. There was a large mass there just as Mr. Thompson had observed, but it was not cancerous. It was Silver's urinary bladder stretched to it's fullest. It was almost the size of a softball.

"Something has to be done before the bladder ruptures," was my comment. "We have to reduce the quantity of urine in the bladder and allow the bladder wall to relax to relieve the tension on it. This process may be painful and it will be best to anesthetize Silver to accomplish this task." The Thompsons agreed with my proposal.

I went out to the Mustang and returned to the hospital with my anesthetic machine. I asked the Thompsons to bring Silver with them and we all proceeded to the treatment room. Mr. Thompson extended Silver's right front leg. I located a vein and slowly injected surital as Silver relaxed until he was prone upon the table. Silver was intubated and connected to the machine. I then regulated the amount of gas to accommodate him.

I suggested that the Thompsons wait in the reception room while I back flushed the sediment in the urethra into the bladder to alleviate the blockage. They obliged. I tried several times to clear the passage by back flushing but to no avail. I went out front and explained the situation to the Thompsons and told them I planned to take some X rays to delineate the blockage better. The radiographs revealed a series of small bladder stones lodged in a row just anterior to the bony portion of the penis. The bladder also contained numerous gravel-size particles like those found in the urethra. I remarked that this problem would likely recur as Silver seemed to be predisposed to forming these stones. I went ahead and performed a urethrotomy and cleared the stones amid a gusher of urine being expelled. I removed the catheter that had been placed in the penis and inserted it directly through the incision I made in the urethra. More urine was expelled along with fine sediment.

I broke surgical sterility and returned to the front of the hospital to talk further with the Thompsons. I suggested a urethrostomy, which is a surgery that relocates the urethra to the rear end of a male dog. Future small stones would not be restricted as they now had. I explained that the urethra is soft tissue and will expand to allow stones to pass but when the stones reach the bony penis, no expansion occurs and the blockage results. We discussed the pros and cons of surgery and in the end they agreed that the surgery I had suggested made sense.

After they went home for the evening, I put on sterile gloves again and went back into surgery. An hour later I had completed the urethrostomy and removed my gloves for the last time that evening. A catheter was left in place to insure that the passage of urine could occur without Silver needing to strain to eliminate it.

While the pack that had been put into the autoclave was sterilizing, I called the Thompsons regarding the surgery. After spending time responding to a multitude of questions, I heard the bell go off and excused myself to vent the autoclave. They thanked me for spending post-surgery time with them. I said that if they had any more questions to be sure and ask their regular doctor when they called the hospital in the morning.

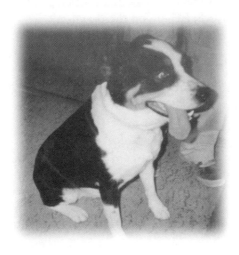

# -49-

## A CANINE SWEATER

**A**fter my hospital closed for the weekend on Saturday, I decided to stay for awhile and hose down the parking lot. I was halfway through this task when a car pulled into the driveway and parked near me. The driver exited his car and walked over and asked if the hospital was still open. I replied in the affirmative and suggested that he go in. I said I was certain that the doctor was somewhere on the premises.

The gentleman entered the hospital with a champagne colored poodle in his arms. I turned off the hose and entered via the rear door. As I put on my smock, I heard the bell on the front counter ring that indicated a client was in the reception room and desired service. I walked into the front office and stood across the counter from the client and his pet. He looked at me for a bit and finally said, "I can see why you were so positive that a doctor was still on the premises." I picked up a blank client/patient card to record the pertinent data that would be forthcoming.

Mr. Alexander gave his name, address, and other information. This male poodle's name was Frisco. Frisco was five years old and had a skin problem. Mr. Alexander was frustrated about the way the groomer trimmed his pet so be bought clippers with the appropriate clipper heads and decided to trim Frisco himself. From a distance, Frisco's coat and grooming pattern looked very good but up close, much was to be desired. Mr. Alexander said, "This is the second time I clipped Frisco. I

208

think that I did a fair job on the coat pattern, but I irritated his skin and now he is chewing at those places where I trimmed him too closely."

We went into the exam room and under better light, it was easy to see the clipper burn or rash where the coat pattern was close to his skin. I told Mr. Alexander that it would heal in a short time if Frisco would leave it alone. On one spot right in the middle of his lower back, Frisco had chewed himself so much that the area was moist and forming a hotspot. I rubbed in a medicated salve with a vanishing cream base that would ease his discomfort. Then I gave him an antibiotic to avoid an infection and a cortisone injection to decrease the skin sensitivity.

Mr. Alexander was fearful that Frisco would continue to chew and scratch at the clipper burns because of habit alone. I agreed that it was possible. To assist in the projected problem, I cut about eighteen inches of four-inch stockingette (tubular gauze) from a roll and using it as a sleeve, put it around Frisco's abdomen. To keep either end in place, I secured it with tape. We both chuckled at the new white sweater that Frisco was sporting.

I asked Mr. Alexander to keep the sweater on Frisco for five to six days. In case Frisco got the one that I had placed on him dirty, I sent home another piece of the roller gauze and tape to secure it. I showed Mr. Alexander a plastic collar but we both agreed that the stockingette was preferred in this case. Mr. Alexander said that he would tell his wife that he had just bought a new sweater for Frisco and that she would have to wait until next year to buy a new one for herself.

I got home just in time to take a call from the Torrance hospital. They patched me through immediately to the Dinsmores. "Archie, our female Beagle, has been sneezing since last night and now she is sneezing so violently that her nose is bleeding. We have had to confine her to the yard to protect our furniture and carpet."

I suggested that they should bring her to the hospital so I could determine what was wrong. "Isn't there anything we can do at home? If we put her in the car, we will have blood all over the interior." I said that they should hold Archie securely in their arms and put an old pillowcase over her head. This should enable them to keep the car clean. They agreed to meet me at the hospital in an hour.

We arrived at the same time—both Dinsmores plus a masked Beagle. I decided to take them directly into the treatment room. Archie had not sneezed at the hospital as yet so I removed the pillowcase to take a better look. I used the cone on the otoscope to do a nasal exam. So much blood was now in both nostrils that neither the Dinsmores nor I knew which nares was involved. I checked the left side first and cleaned it with a cotton swab. Nothing significant was noted. I became rather bold in my technique and placed the cone in the right nostril. This caused Archie to sneeze. The lens on the otoscope was of no further use as it was covered with blood. My glasses were in the same condition. My forehead, chin, and smock were decorated with blood spots. I decided to use another approach.

I administered surital in the vein and added demerol to suppress the sneezing reflex. Next I passed an endotracheal tube to divert her breathing through it rather than through her nostrils. Using cotton-tipped applicators, I cleaned out all of the frank blood from both nares. Now I was ready to reexamine her. Again I started with the left side—nothing. The right nostril was still bleeding slightly. I could swab out the blood and then quickly take a peak with the otoscope before further bleeding obliterated my view. Four or five peeks later I still had not found anything and I was about to give up, but the condition of that nostril made me suspicious that something was there.

I decided to look one more time and, this time, I located a foxtail lodged deep in the soft tissue. I grasped the awns and attempted to remove it, but the awns broke off. After several attempts, I was able to grip the body of the foxtail and remove it. I packed the nares because it was bleeding more profusely than before. I told the Dinsmores that they could take Archie home. They looked at each other. Finally Mrs. Dinsmore said, "Can we leave him here? She will only cause more damage at home if she continues to sneeze. If you put her in a cage at least the area of damage will be much smaller. Besides, Archie will need a bath to remove all of the blood on her. We would be able to pick her up tomorrow sometime after her bath." I said that would be fine. "What do you suggest we clean up our carpet and furniture with?" I suggested using hydrogen peroxide as that is what I use to clean slacks, shirts, and smocks when they are blood stained. I feel that it would be safe to use on carpets and upholstery. All of us stopped at the sink and washed our hands and faces. Mrs. Dinsmore suggested that I look in a mirror as I still had numerous red freckles on my face.

It was dusk when Dick Hyde phoned through the Manhattan Beach exchange. He had just returned from a pheasant hunting trip in northern

California. I had met him on occasion at social events and whenever we got to visiting, all he would talk about was his English Setter, Corker. Dick had invested considerable money in having Corker trained for bird hunting and would always expound on his dog's attributes.

I was greeted with a "Hi doc, Corker's got a problem." I inquired as to what the problem might be and he said that his Setter had raw spots under each eye that were really bothering him. I agreed to meet him at the hospital and left immediately. Dick had Corker on a leash and was walking him in the parking lot when I arrived. We went into the exam room and I was able to get a much better look at two pronounced raw areas—one under each eye. I inquired as to what might cause such an unusual bilateral injury and Dick said, "We were pheasant hunting in a harvested rice field. The birds had sought cover in the rice checks where there was protection. That area is overgrown with weeds, light brush, and rice that has lodged. Corker goes into these places to flush the birds and he parts the underbrush with his nose. The sores are a result of this action."

I treated the raw spots with salve and told Dick that they were going to have to heal on their own. I did make him aware of the fact that it would happen again under similar circumstances and the injury would be worse each time it happened. This worried him. Corker could not flush the pheasants without getting into the rice checks.

Dick said that Corker needed a helmet and visor just like the knights of old. That gave me an idea. I thought that if soft chamois was fitted over Corker's head and holes were cut into it for vision, that possibly Corker could avoid repetitious injuries.

Two weeks later, Dick stopped by my office with Corker. Corker had on a black chamois "mask" that was fitted to protect his face. Dick said, "Corker has on the Mask of Zorro." The Setter didn't seem to mind the headpiece and from the looks of the way it was styled to fit his head, I felt that it would give him excellent protection. I agreed with Dick that Corker should not go out again in the rice fields to hunt birds anymore this year. However, I felt that if they hunted in cotton or other fields of that nature, Corker could hunt without causing further injury to his face.

# —50—

# A TORTOISE CASE

I was listening to the boys' prayers when I heard the phone ring. When I turned around, Marna was in the bedroom doorway motioning to me that I should attend to the incoming phone call. The operator informed me that Mr. Freeholtz had explained to her what needed to be done and wanted to talk to a doctor that could help them. She said, "I'll let Mr. Freeholtz explain the problem to you."

Mr Freeholtz was patched through and he asked me to just be a sounding board while he dumped a sad request on me. Their Airdale, Rusty, was eighteen years old and had been failing for the past two years. Now Rusty could hardly walk, and this morning he started expelling bloody diarrhea.

"I know that he should be put to sleep but Rusty belongs to my daughter who is away at college. She knows Rusty is failing but she made us promise that we would not have him put to sleep. Now Rusty has lived out his life and the end must be hastened. If Rusty dies at a hospital, my daughter will certainly call and ask how he died. Can you help me with this situation?"

I was really in a bind. I simply refused to lie to his daughter if she called, and on the other hand, something humane needed to be done to alleviate Rusty's pain and suffering. Several moments passed and then I suggested that he bring Rusty down to the hospital and I would euthanize him. If his daughter did call, I would tell her that Rusty died at the hospital as the result of old age and other problems.

Both Mr. and Mrs. Freeholtz arrived at my Redondo Beach hospital forty minutes later. Both had been crying and the first thing they said was that if Becky ever found out, she would probably never forgive them. Rusty was a stenchy mess. Because he was too weak to stand, the bloody diarrhea was smeared all over his rear end. They had brought Rusty into the hospital wrapped in a beach towel. We went together into the treatment room and I performed the requested task. I entered on the patient card, "Died at hospital of old age and other problems." We shook hands and they left after squaring up the account.

When I left for home, they were still in the parking lot trying to convince themselves that they had done the right thing. I walked over to their car and tried to comfort them. They informed me that Becky was one year old when they bought Rusty for a birthday gift. "When Becky left for college, she really mourned for her life-long companion. Becky would call home and ask to talk to Rusty. We would hold the phone to Rusty's ear and Becky would say, 'speak' and Rusty would answer with a 'woof'! Becky and Rusty were inseparable friends." I watched them slowly pull out of the parking lot and sympathized with the decision that had confronted them.

The next morning I made an additional note on the patient card asking Jo to let me handle any phone calls from Becky Freeholtz. A few days passed, then a week, then several weeks. We never had to respond to Becky's anticipated phone call. I was relieved.

The sky was just lighting up in the east as I pulled out of the driveway. I decided to stop and return to the house for my shaving kit because there was a definite possibility that after this case, I might go directly to my practice for my morning's schedule. Little traffic was on the road as I headed for the Lawndale practice. The clients were in their car waiting when I arrived. The morning air was crisp and refreshed my senses as I walked over and tapped on the fogged-up window of their car to indicate that I had arrived.

The Brinkmans escorted their Labrador, Barbie, into the exam room, and I checked her swollen foot. I gently manipulated the foot and noted it was very painful as Barbie objected and tried to pull it from my grasp. When I rotated the toes on her injured right fore foot, she cried in discomfort. I recommended an X ray and the Brinkmans readily agreed that it was a good idea. Fifteen minutes later all three of us were scanning the radiograph on the view screen. It was very evident that there were three distinct fractures—one each on three of her metacarpal bones.

I had given Barbie an intramuscular sedative injection a little earlier and it was beginning to take effect. This allowed me to fit a comfortable walking splint to her paw in order to protect the foot from further damage from the sharp ends of the fragmented bones. When all was done, I carried Barbie into the pre-surgery ward and tucked her into a cage. I explained to the Brinkmans that in a little over an hour their regular veterinarian would be on the premises and that Barbie would then be in his care. I suggested that they call the hospital in about a half an hour when the hospital opened. This would be ample time for the doctor to evaluate the films that I had taken. Then he would be able to explain a course of action involving the fracture repairs.

As the Brinkmans left, I glanced at my watch. I returned the hospital to its original state and then decided to have breakfast at a local restaurant before heading to my hospital where I planned to clean up and shave to make myself presentable for my morning's first client.

As I pulled into my hospital's parking lot, a client was waiting for my arrival. They were delighted that I was early for they had a tortoise that was injured. Somehow the Flores's tortoise, Pokey, had escaped the confines of their yard and been hit or run over in the street. Mr. Flores had found Pokey near the curb when he went outside to bring in the morning paper. I checked Pokey over and he seemed to be in pretty good shape despite a crack in his shell that was rather extensive. I had no knowledge on how to treat this type of injury so I picked up the phone and called a colleague that was more proficient in this type of case. After several minutes on the phone, I returned to the exam room and explained what needed to be done. Pokey's shell needed to be stabilized and then sealed so that he would not dehydrate. They left Pokey in my care and were just exiting the hospital when Jo arrived.

I asked Jo to go down the street to the local drug store and purchase several candles—preferably white ones. In the meantime I located a bit and the proper size drill plus the heaviest stainless steel surgical suture material I could find. I then sterilized the wire and was ready when Jo returned with some white candles. I had all the necessary equipment at hand now and was ready to proceed with Jo's assistance.

Jo restrained Pokey and I drilled a series of holes an inch apart on either side of the cracked shell. I then carefully wired the shells together, being very careful not to penetrate the shell too deeply. Jo then heated the candle wax, and warm wax was used to seal the shell. A warm spatula was used to smear the wax over the shell so that the entire shell was now completely sealed. We both stood back and admired the job.

Jo and I were still talking about our tortoise case as we walked to the front desk and met our first regular client of the day. She looked at my unshaven face and said, "You look as if you have been up all night!"

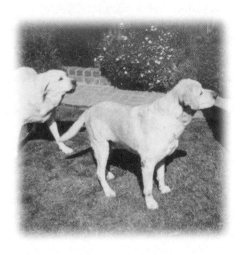

# -51-

## TIME OUT!

**I**t was the Tuesday after Labor Day, and Jo told me that Marna had called for me to be ready to go to lunch with her. All of my morning clients had been dispatched and two sterility surgeries completed when Marna stepped into my office.

I told Jo that I would be back in an hour. Marna said, "Two!" We had a leisurely lunch at a nice restaurant. Marna told me that I was working too many hours—all day at my own hospital and most of the rest of the time elsewhere taking emergencies for my colleagues. "I want to spend more time with you and I do need help raising our sons!" was her mandate. "You just have to slow down. I want you to take off a day a week from your office. This will not effect your emergency contracts since you will only be gone during the day. How about taking Thursdays off?" I said that it would probably be a good idea but that I couldn't implement it for a couple of weeks because of the appointments already scheduled. "Honey," she said, "I have already worked it out with Jo. You have no Thursday appointments for the entire month. Take a time out!" Marna was insistent, so I complied with her request.

When I got back to the office, Jo was all smiles. She and Marna had been planning this for some time and I was completely unaware of their scheming. I knew my vigorous routing was putting a strain on me, but I had failed to assess how it was effecting Marna and the boys. I now could look forward to Thursdays as my day of relaxation in the middle

216

of the week. As I drove home that evening, I mulled over the after-noon's conversation in my mind. I guess that I was trying to figure out how to manage all of this time off. I walked into the house while pondering the luxury of having Thursdays off when the spell was broken as the phone rang.

Marna handed me the phone. She had a smile on her face and blew me a kiss as I put the receiver to my ear. I knew what she was thinking, but now I had to concentrate on the telephone conversation. The Manhattan Beach operator had a party on the line who called about a dog that was limping. I was informed that the party did not wish to bring the dog in on an emergency but just needed to obtain some advice as how to care for their pet until their regular doctor's hospital opened in the morning.

I was on the phone several minutes and when I hung up, Marna asked where I was off to now? I told her that I did not have to respond to that call other than give advice. Marna was smiling.

It was just about bedtime when I picked up the receiver. The San Pedro operator informed me that Mrs. Simpson wanted me to see her injured cat. Mrs. Simpson was crying so I had difficulty understanding what the problem was, but I did manage to convey when and where to meet me before she hung up, as well as for her to leave for that loca-tion as soon as possible. Mrs. Simpson arrived before me and she was hysterical. Pojo, her yellow Tabby cat, was a bloody mess. Pojo was vomiting foamy blood mixed with hair. I asked Mrs. Simpson to place the cat carrier on the exam table and then suggested that she sit down. She complied.

I extracted Pojo from his cage and was surprised how strong he appeared to be despite the apparent considerable loss of blood. I found only a small laceration at the side of Pojo's neck and it had been bleeding profusely but the hemorrhaging had almost completely stoped by this time. I was certain there were more lesions so I carefully went over the matted bloody coat with careful inspection. No more wounds were noted. Pojo seemed to be alert so I plunked him into the tub and carefully washed his fur expecting to find other lesions that I had not previously located. Again, none were found.

During the bathing process, clotted blood was expelled from the wound on his neck so I asked Mrs. Simpson to hold Pojo while I went to the Mustang for my anesthetic machine. Soon Pojo was under anesthesia.

I took him into surgery after assuring Mrs. Simpson that most of the blood loss, which appeared to be minimal, was spread over a large area of Pojo's body making it appear that he had hemorrhaged much more.

I was able to locate the severed vessel and tied it off. I then cleaned the wound and sutured the laceration. I could hear the phone ringing. I looked up at the clock and it was a few minutes past one in the morning. I looked at the telephone and the call was coming in on the hospital's backline. I could not get to the phone right away to see who was calling but I knew if it was Marna, the phone would ring again in four minutes. It did. As soon as I was finished with surgery and took off my gloves, I called home.

There was a call from the Hawthorne exchange about a Pekinese in whelp. The operator had left the client's phone number so I was able to call directly. Mrs. Blaymore answered and thanked me for calling so promptly. Blondie had delivered one pup but that was all. Another pup was partially exposed but could not be delivered. Mrs. Blaymore said, "Both my husband and I think Blondie should be seen by you. We are almost certain that the pup she is now trying to deliver is dead." I told them I could meet them at the Hawthorne hospital and for them to leave right away.

I prepared a recovery cage for Pojo and placed him in it, said good-night to Mrs. Simpson as she left, washed up and headed for Hawthorne. I knew that I would have to return and clean up the hospital before my night's work was completed.

Blondie was wrapped up in a blanket carried by Mr. Blaymore. Mrs. Blaymore had the newborn pup in a padded basket and followed her husband in. We went directly to the treatment room for the initial exami-nation. The situation was exactly as described and the pup retained in the birth canal was indeed dead. It was an extra large pup and swollen beside. There was little chance that it could have been delivered normally and consequently would require some help. I decided to attempt an instrument delivery so I blocked the area with the local anesthetic, xylocaine.

While the anesthetic was taking effect, I got all of the instruments ready. I then put on surgical gloves and went to work commencing with an episiotomy incision. With a little tug from me and a push by Blondie, the dead pup was delivered. I now realized why Blondie had so much trouble giving birth for this pup was badly deformed. By this time Blondie was exhausted and needed help in delivering the rest of her litter.

Mr. Blaymore continued to hold his pet and Mrs. Blaymore held Blondie's right front leg while I administered the hormone oxytocin. Blondie began straining almost immediately, and in a few minutes, two more healthy pups joined their siblings in the basket.

I closed the episiotomy incision with a couple of sutures and we journeyed as a group to the reception room. Mrs. Blaymore sat down in a chair and started crying. Her husband comforted her. Finally she said, "I was afraid that we were going to lose Blondie." I assured her that all was well now and that the large misshapened pup had caused all of the problem. We took another look at the basket of three. Blondie was very attentive so I suggested that they head for home and allow the pups to dine for the first time.

I hurriedly cleaned up the hospital and returned to San Pedro and cleaned up that hospital's surgery room before calling it a night.

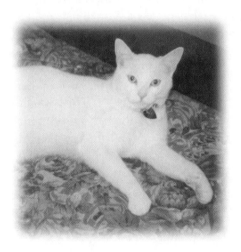

—————————/\\————————————**52-**

# AVOCADO PITS

**C**romwell was standing in the examination room beside me. I was contemplating how I would get him up on the exam table with only the two owners and myself to lift him. Cromwell had been a long-time patient of mine and I knew what he weighed—fifteen more pounds that myself. He was not a large St. Bernard—he was an immense St. Bernard.

I remembered the time Mrs. Berger asked me how to get Cromwell to stand on the scales so she could weigh him. I remarked that she was approaching the problem wrong. "All you have to do is hold Cromwell in your arms and then step on the scales. Then weigh only yourself. The difference is Cromwell's weight." She had glared at me and said, "Got any other stupid suggestions?" We both laughed at the problems we faced with Cromwell's size.

The Bergers had called my hospital's exchange because Cromwell had been vomiting off and on for several days. There did not appear to be any pattern to his problem. Sometime vomiting occurred an hour or so after a meal and then on other occasions maybe a day or two apart. Mrs. Berger said, "I normally had the task of cleaning up the mess in the house, but last night I was out and my husband had the job of cleaning up the carpet. Ken said to get to the bottom of the problem or confine Cromwell to the yard because this is the last time I will clean up after him! If that happened, being banished from the house would break Cromwell's heart."

220

We got Cromwell to stand and then Mr. Berger and I locked hands underneath his abdomen and lifted Cromwell up on the table. The Bergers kept a tight leash on him, holding it snugly so he would not try to jump to the floor. All of Cromwell's vital signs were normal. However, as my examination progressed, I was able to palpate two large masses in his stomach. One was about twice the size of the other. With this information in mind, I tried to explain to the owners what I thought was causing their pet to vomit irregularly. "These objects were occasionally blocking the pylorus, the exit of the stomach and the entrance to the bowel. If and when this blockage occurred, any ingesta in the stomach might backup and be expelled orally.

I suggested that I give Cromwell some apomorphine to make him vomit more violently. Hopefully he would be able to expel these masses orally. After all, he did ingest them so returning them to the outside world was a definite possibility. Apomorphine was given and Cromwell performed superbly. I held a large waste basket and he disgorged his last meal in a splendid fashion. After the emetic had accomplished the desired effect and the waste basket was half full, I took basket and contents to the rear of the hospital to inspect what Cromwell had passed. I soon located a round object and took it over to the sink to rinse it off to facilitate identification. It appeared to be a ball, but I was wrong. It was an avocado seed about the size of a ping-pong ball. I dried it off and took it back to the exam room to show the Bergers.

Mrs. Berger said, "When I let Cromwell out in the morning, he uses the corner of our yard as a toilet and then goes over to our neighbor's yard and checks to see if any avocados have dropped during the night. He makes this trip daily He sometimes brings them back into our yard, peels them carefully before devouring the fleshy part. I have never known him to ingest a seed but the seeds can be slippery. I guess if the circumstances are right, he could accidentally swallow one."

While this explanation was going on, I was again palpating the St. Bernard's abdomen. I could only feel one mass in his stomach—he had expelled the smaller of the two. I said that the larger seed may be too large to exit via vomition. "Since we don't know if one seed, the other seed, or both caused the problem, I have no idea if the situation has been corrected or not," I said. The Bergers spoke quietly to each other for a few minutes and then turned and asked me, "Are you suggesting that surgery might be the answer?" I responded in the affirmative. They agreed with my proposal.

Now I was confronted with a surgery case on a dog that was larger than I. I was concerned on how to physically handle my patient. Mr. Berger volunteered to help me get Cromwell into surgery and I readily accepted his help. I brought in my anesthetic machine and took it into surgery. That task was very easy. My next effort would involve locating my patient on the surgery table.

I gave Cromwell a surital sedative intravenously in the exam room so he would be easier for us to handle. He settled gently on the table and the Bergers situated themselves on either side of the table so he would not fall off. I then rolled in my gurney and we slid Cromwell over on it. As we went through the doorways, we had to flex his legs to enable us to make passage. The gurney was placed next to the surgery table and Cromwell was moved over on it. The thoracic positioners on the table were raised on either side and our patient was on his back in a cradle-like manner so there was no way that he could roll off. I connected the anesthetic machine to the largest endotracheal tube I had and then inflated the cuff so that all the metafane gas I gave to him would be efficiently used to maintain the proper level of anesthetic.

I suggested they return home as I would be in surgery for awhile. As soon as they left, I called Marna and requested assistance. She arrived with all three boys while I was in surgery. It did not take long to locate the avocado seed and I positioned it between the feathered edges of converging capillaries and made an incision that would be large enough to remove the foreign body. Soon the large avocado seed was on display on the mayo tray and I was closing the gastrostomy incision. The skin incision was closed next and moments later I took off my surgical gloves and gown. I looked at this giant dog. Cromwell was longer than my five-foot surgery table. His head was resting on my second mayo tray and his feet extended a good two feet or more past the other end of the table.

Marna, Allen, and I struggled to get a protective bodywrap around Cromwell's middle. It took five rolls of four-inch elastic tape to insure that the protective gauze would remain in its proper position. George and Albert had prepared a cage while the bandage was being applied to Cromwell. Now we were faced with the job of removing Cromwell from the table and placing him in his prepared cage. While I was contemplating how to proceed, Allen disconnected the anesthetic machine and rolled it out to the Mustang.

When Allen returned, I explained to the family how I intended to implement my plan. We located a large blanket and then passed it under Cromwell's body. It took a lot of effort. Next we dropped the hydraulic surgery table to its lowest position and tilted it. With Albert watching and Marna and Allen on one side and George and I one the other, we allowed Cromwell to gently slide off the table onto the floor. We then used the blanket as a sled and dragged him into the ward and rolled him over into his cage. We had to bend his legs to close the cage doors. When he woke up, he would be able to stand but he might have difficulty turning around in his cage. It was going to be in his best interest to discharge him early the next morning.

Marna remarked that she hadn't started dinner yet. In fact, she hadn't decided what to fix either. I was aware that she was indirectly fishing for an invitation to go out to dinner. Everyone was happy when I suggested eating at a local restaurant. Marna volunteered to look up the telephone number of the restaurant that I had selected and then call the answering services so they would know my location. Allen had already started cleaning the surgical instruments and George and Albert were busy cleaning the surgery room. I asked Albert to wash off the avocado seed so I could show it to the Bergers in the morning. I spent time completing the paper work. With so many of us helping out, the work was quickly completed.

Thirty minutes later we were looking at a menu and trying to decide what would satisfy our tastes. Our conversation was soon involved with the largest dog that I had ever seen, treated, or had in surgery. Cromwell was by far the largest dog that I had ever had on a surgery table and probably he tied for first or second in the other two categories.

Marna and the younger two boys headed home and Allen returned to the hospital with me to check on Cromwell. Allen vented the autoclave while I went into the ward. I returned to get the Berger's phone number from the patient card and just sat by the phone thinking. I had just completed surgery on an animal that was larger than most humans, but I was glad I had chosen the veterinary medical profession rather than becoming a physician. Cromwell was now beginning to wake up so I picked up the phone and dialed the Bergers to give them the post-surgery report.

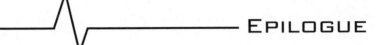

**I**t was a few minutes past midnight on the morning of August 29, 1974. As I drove west to Palos Verdes, I wondered if this would be the last off-hours emergency that I would take. It was! The only emergencies I would take in the future would be during regular office hours at my own hospital.

This change in my life commenced in 1972 when I was growing weary of working days and part of each night with only a few hours of sleep. My own hospital was growing and demanding more attention. My family was growing also. I realized that my three sons were no longer children but young men. They needed the assistance of a father to help their mother rear them in a manner that would be pleasing to both man and God.

In 1972, I talked with the eleven hospitals about giving up taking their emergencies. Several new hospitals had opened in the area and they also wanted emergency coverage. With these thoughts in mind, a group of over eighty veterinarians met one afternoon at a restaurant to find a way to solve their concerns. A committee of five was appointed to find a solution. I was one of those five. This committee became the original board when it was incorporated under the name of Emergency Pet Clinic of South Bay, Inc. (EPC). Thirty-five veterinarians funded this new corporation and became the original shareholders.

A building in Torrance was leased and at six o'clock in the evening on August 29 1974, the EPC opened its doors for the first time. This was the

225

Friday night of Labor Day weekend and the EPC started business with a boom and has been busy ever since. The EPC's success has continued over its twenty-five year existence. The current board consists of my colleagues Teresa Benton, Frank Dieter, Robert Streeter, Richard Sullivan, and myself. With the advice and assistance of Robert Hyman of the accounting firm Diversified Veterinary Management, we have overcome numerous obstacles but have continued to grow and provide the services that are needed in the field of veterinary emergency medicine in the community.

The EPC is more prone to be described as an emergency referral practice with a heavy emphasis on "referral." Cases taken in are treated for emergency problems only and then referred back to the hospital that sent them. This way the original hospital provides the further treatment and aftercare.

Veterinary facilities in the area can also send critical cases to the EPC for them to monitor overnight or over the weekend since there is always a veterinarian and staff on duty during the hours they are open. The doctor on duty is backed up by a qualified lay staff to enable the EPC to provide the very best care possible.

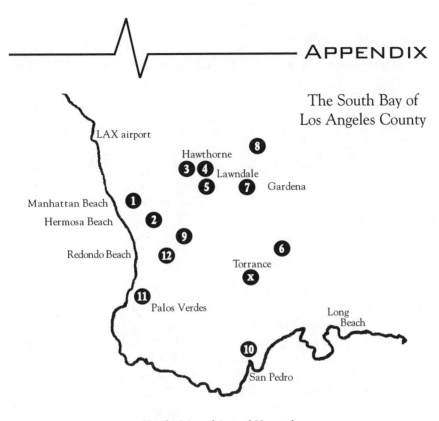

The South Bay of
Los Angeles County

Key for Map of Animal Hospitals

1. Bay Air Animal Hospital, Manhattan Beach
2. Hermosa Beach Animal Hospital, Hermosa Beach
3. Hollypark Animal Hospital, Hawthorne
4. Hawthorne Animal Hospital, Hawthorne
5. Lawndale Pet Hospital, Lawndale
6. Harbor Animal Hospital, Torrance
7. Alondra Animal Hospital, Gardena
8. Inland Animal Hospital, Gardena
9. Redwood Animal Hospital, Redondo Beach
10. San Pedro Animal Hospital, San Pedro
11. Palos Verdes Animal Hospital, Palos Verdes*
12. Marina Animal Hospital, Redondo Beach**
x. Home (Torrance)

*Actually in Redondo Beach
**My hospital—opened June 22, 1970

# ABOUT THE AUTHOR

George Albert Porter attended the University of California at Davis where he received a bachelor of science in animal husbandry in 1952, specializing in animal nutrition.

After operating a family farm in Indiana for a year, he was drafted into the army and served in the infantry in Korea for two years. Upon his discharge, he returned to farming and married Marilyn Bradley of Redondo Beach, California, in 1956. In 1957, he decided to return to school, attending Stanford University. He then graduated from the School of Veterinary Medicine at UCD in 1962.

He opened his own practice, Marina Animal Hospital, in 1970 in Redondo Beach and practiced there until 1990 when he retired as a clinician.

Porter served as president of the Torrance Rotary Club 1968–69. In 1972 he was appointed by his colleagues to be on a committee to explore the possibilities of establishing an emergency pet hospital to serve the many veterinary clinics in the area. This practice, the Emergency Pet Clinic of South Bay, Inc., was an immediate success. Porter has served on the board of directors since its inception.

In 1997 Porter and his wife, Marilyn, moved to Santa Barbara, California, for retirement. While there, he was inspired to compile a series of events from his veterinary career. *Pet ER* and *ER Vet* are the results of his efforts.